# Chondromalacia of the Patella

# Chondromalacia of the Patella

Editors
## Justus C. Pickett, M.D.
*Professor Emeritus*
*Department of Orthopedic Surgery*
*School of Medicine*
*West Virginia University*
*Morgantown, West Virginia*

## Eric L. Radin, M.D.
*Professor and Chairman*
*Department of Orthopedic Surgery*
*School of Medicine*
*West Virginia University*
*Morgantown, West Virginia*

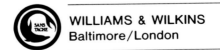
**WILLIAMS & WILKINS**
Baltimore/London

Copyright © 1983
William & Wilkins
428 East Preston Street
Baltimore, MD 21202, U.S.A.

*Made in the United States of America*

**Library of Congress Cataloging in Publication Data**

Main entry under title:

Chondromalacia of the patella.

Includes index.
1. Chondromalacia patellae. I. Pickett, Justus C. II. Radin, Eric L. [DNLM: 1.
Patella—Congresses. 2. Cartilage diseases—Etiology—Congresses. 3. Cartilage dis-
eases—Therapy—Congresses. WE 870 C548 1981]
RC935.C48C48 1983        617'.582        83-7036
ISBN 0-683-06877-6

Composed and printed at the
Waverly Press, Inc.
Mt. Royal and Guilford Aves.
Baltimore, MD 21202, U.S.A.

# Preface

Chondromalacia of the patella is the most common diagnosis made for pain in the knee. In spite of the widespread incidence, it remains one of the most confusing and enigmatic problems to those who treat musculoskeletal conditions. There seems to be no relationship between the symptoms and the pathological finding of softening and fibrillation of the articular cartilage of the underside of the patella inasmuch as these changes are commonly reported as incidental observations in arthroscopic and surgical explorations of the knee for other pathological entities. At autopsy, such findings are almost universal with age, even though pain under the knee cap is not totally ubiquitous. The epidemiology of chondromalacia of the patella is also confusing in that a peak occurs in young adolescent girls and again in later life as a concomitant finding associated with osteoarthrosis and deterioration of the femorotibial joint in older age. There is also no reliable cure and what treatments there are frequently make no sense. The majority of young adolescent females with pain in the patellofemoral joint respond well to progressive resistance strengthening exercises of the quadriceps which obviously squeeze the patella into the femoral groove! Total excision of the patella, which should obviously relieve any symptoms originating from the patella, in a significant number of cases often fails to relieve the symptoms. Chondral shaving, lateral release, muscle realignment, tibial tubercle reimplantation, and even just simple arthroscopic lavage all work in some patients but it is almost impossible to predict in which patients.

Very recently, a more sensible approach to the etiology and treatment of chondromalacia of the patella seems to be emerging. The stimulus for this understanding has primarily come from those investigators trying to understand how joints wear out. It is only in the last several years that relationships are beginning to emerge between the biological degradation of joint tissues and alterations in the mechanical stress to which these tissues are subjected. The long held belief that articular cartilage fibrillation must progress has been shown to be a myth. These investigators have been interested in the patella because of its accessability, relatively small size, and the observation that progressive and nonprogressive cartilage fibrillation frequently exist within 1 cm or less on the articular surface of this bone. This intense study of the patella and the patellofemoral joint has finally begun to point the way to an understanding of the etiology and a rational basis for the treatment of chondromalacia of the patella.

The events leading to this understanding were occuring in widely separate laboratories and clinics throughout the world and the findings, because they were emerging from multiple disciplines, were frequently not fully known by all interested parties. Several investigators in this field simultaneously felt the need to gather together to discuss the progress to date and the directions for future experimental and clinical research in this area. It was clear that, up to the point of this Symposium, there were features of many of the key works that had much more in common than their published and presented versions would indicate, simply because all were not using the same terms and were frequently approaching identical problems with a different perspective and outlook. It was believed that if the key authorities in this field had the opportunity to discuss chondromalacia in depth, that some sense of common understanding of the condition would emerge. The purpose, therefore, of this *Symposium of the Etiology and Treatment of Chondromalacia of the Patella* was to find areas of agreement regarding the etiology, to discover what the meaningful but as yet unanswered questions about what the causes of chondromalacia were, and to define clearly a rational approach for the treatment of this condition. The Symposium was difficult to arrange because, rather than just identifying a group of suitable speakers, the organizers had to bring particular individuals together under one roof at one time. Since all of those who participated have international reputations, and commitments frequently scheduled years in advance, it was a very difficult task, not made any easier by the fact that the participants came from several different countries. It was clear, however, that the purpose of the symposium would be unfulfilled if even one of the key individuals could not participate, as the goal was not only to make a status report but also to point out the way to the future.

It finally happened in Morgantown, in June of 1981. It took some extraordinary juggling of the schedules and for several, some unorthodox travel arrangements.

The beauty of the Symposium was not only that it included all of the major figures whose recent contributions were leading in new directions, but it also allowed full discussion between the participants. These discussions occurred during the formal Symposium sessions and in private. Fortunately, the proceedings were recorded and what has emerged was what was hoped for: namely, an understanding of the etiology and a rational basis for treatment of chondromalacia of the patella. This volume contains the formal presentations of the participants, the discussions among themselves, the answers to questions from the audience of over 200 orthopaedic surgeons and rheumatologists. In retrospect, the Symposium was a watershed. Although all of the questions regarding the etiology and treatment of chondromalacia of the patella are not answered, chondromalacia need no longer be considered a mystery and treatment can be carried out on a rational basis. The Symposium was truly a remarkable orthopaedic and rheumatological event and it is quite reasonable to expect that the concepts enunciated at this Symposium will be the framework on which the medical community can, for the first time, now logically build a construct for an understanding of what was once one of the major orthopaedic enigmas of our time.

We wish to acknowledge the help from the West Virginia University Department of Orthopedic Surgery Orthopedic Education and Research Fund and the West Virginia University Department of the Continuing Medical Education in the development of this Symposium.

It is appropriate, at this time, for the organizers to express their gratitude to the participants who appreciated the unique significance of this Symposium and participated, for the entire 2 days, with enthusiasm and true intellectual honesty. We must also thank the University of West Virginia School of Medicine and the commercial donors who sponsored the Symposium. Our thanks should also be given to Williams & Wilkins, whose medical editors understood the importance of this meeting and allowed these proceedings to be published in their entirety, in order that this "happening" be preserved for posterity.

Justus C. Pickett, M.D.                                    Eric L. Radin, M.D.

# Contributors

**Ward Casscells, M.D.**
Attending Chief of Orthopaedics, Wilmington Medical Center and St. Francis Hospital, Consultant, Alfred I. Dupont Institute, Wilmington, Delaware

**Paul Ficat, M.D.**
Professor Agrege, Universite Paul Sabatier, Toulouse, France

**John Goodfellow, M.S., F.R.C.S.**
Professor of Orthopaedics, The Nuffield Orthopaedic Centre, Headington, Oxford, England

**David S. Hungerford, M.D.**
Associate Professor of Orthopedic Surgery, The John Hopkins University, School of Medicine, Baltimore, Maryland

**John Insall, F.R.C.S.**
Professor of Orthopedic Surgery, Cornell University Medical College, Director of Knee Service, Hospital for Joint Diseases, New York, New York

**Carroll Laurin, M.D.**
Professor and Chairman of Orthopedic Surgery, Hotel-Dieu de Montreal Hospital, University of Montreal, Montreal, Canada

**Rudolph Lemperg, M.D., Ph.D.**
Professor, Department of Orthopedic Surgery, School of Medicine, West Virginia University, Morgantown, West Virginia

**Paul Maquet, M.D.**
Professor of Orthopedic Surgery, Awyaille, Belgium

**George Meachim, M.D.**
Professor of Pathology, Department of Pathology, Royal Liverpool Hospital, University of Liverpool, Liverpool, England

**Eric L. Radin, M.D.**
Professor and Chairman, Department of Orthopedic Surgery, School of Medicine, West Virginia University, Morgantown, West Virginia

**Justis C. Pickett, M.D.**
Professor Emeritus, Department of Orthopedic Surgery, School of Medicine, West Virginia University, Morgantown, West Virginia

# Contents

# CHAPTER ONE

# Cartilage Lesions on the Patella

GEORGE MEACHIM, M.D.

A considerable variety of degenerative lesions can occur in patellar articular cartilage. They vary in the methods required for their detection, their morphology, and their potential to progress to full-thickness cartilage loss with bone exposure.

Transmission electron microscopy has shown that one important form of cartilage degeneration is characterized by an abnormally wide separation of the collagen fibers of the intercellular matrix (9). Water content is increased in this abnormality, so that the cartilage feels soft on palpation (i.e., it shows "chondromalacia" in a descriptive sense). Initially, the ultrastructural deterioration in the collagen fiber framework within the cartilage matrix may or may not be accompanied by breaks in the continuity of the cartilage surface, but sooner or later surface fraying and splitting become apparent histologically or by Indian ink staining, and eventually become apparent macroscopically on unstained surfaces. Another sort of histological lesion is seen as tiny horizontal splits at the interface between the uncalcified cartilage matrix and its calcified base (7). This horizontal splitting is attributable to shearing damage. It is debatable whether it is related to ultrastructural deterioration of the collagen fiber framework of the overlying cartilage, or whether it occurs independently. In some instances, these tiny lesions can develop into major shearing splits.

An increase in water content explains the surprising fact that cartilage can be thicker than normal during the early stages of degeneration (6). It also explains why fronds of degenerating patellar cartilage sometimes protrude above the level of the adjacent articular surface.

Further development of degeneration will, of course, eventually lead to thinning of the cartilage from destructive tissue loss

1

(8). One or more of the following lesions are seen in cartilage segments undergoing destructive degeneration (Fig. 1.1):

1. Deep vertical splitting and disintegration of fibrillation type;

2. A grinding down of the cartilage from abrasive wear, without the deep splitting typical of fibrillation;

3. Major horizontal splitting at the interface between calcified and uncalcified cartilage, attributable to shearing damage.

In certain circumstances, cartilage degeneration can progress to complete loss of an area of cartilage, thus giving bone exposure and bone wear of osteoarthritic type. Our studies (3) of the natural history of patellar lesions have shown that fibrillation can be either progressive to bone exposure (i.e., osteoarthritic)

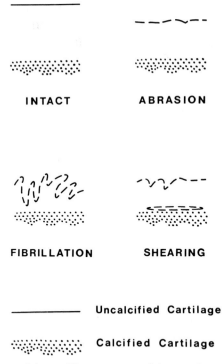

**Figure 1.1.** Diagram of three different types of destructive cartilage lesion. *Fibrillation:* splitting extending obliquely and then vertically into the uncalcified cartilage along the alignments of its collagen fiber framework. *Abrasion:* smoother surfaced destructive thinning. *Shearing:* horizontal splitting along the interface between the uncalcified cartilage and its calcified base. More than one type of destructive lesion can occur in the same cartilage segment.

or of limited progression (i.e., not truly osteoarthritic). The same probably holds true for minor shearing splits. However, abrasive wear and major shearing damage both seem to be strongly associated with an osteoarthritic potential.

The degenerative lesions so far mentioned occur mainly in cartilage which is still exposed to the joint cavity at its synovial interface. In another type of lesion, seen especially at the periphery of the patella, a layer of fibrous tissue, sometimes only one or two cells thick, encroaches over the original cartilage surface.

## INDIAN INK AND HISTOLOGICAL STUDIES OF NECROPSY MATERIAL

A study of patellae from random necropsies in Liverpool has shown that sites of fraying and other lesions of the patella are extremely common in the adult population. Thus, the surface of adult patellar cartilage can be either intact or not intact on histological examination: both states are "normal" in human adults. Milder lesions are not readily apparent to the naked eye, and may require Indian ink staining of the surface or histology for their detection. Using such methods, it can be shown that patellar surface lesions are often already present in young adults, that they first develop at the periphery of the cartilage sheet, and that there is an age-related increase in the percentage of the surface area affected and in the severity of the cartilage damage. In older subjects, a high percentage of the patellar surface may no longer be histologically intact.

## MACROSCOPIC STUDIES OF NECROPSY MATERIAL

In a more recent study of necropsy patellae in Liverpool, we intentionally confined our observations to lesions which were apparent to the naked eye without first staining the surface with Indian ink. This study was designed to record only lesions of the sort likely to be detected visually on surgical exploration of the knee or arthroscopy. We found that such lesions are usually first apparent at a later age and at a different site from those detected with Indian ink. As in the case of the Indian ink lesions, macroscopic lesions again show an age-releated increase in their extent and severity (1).

For this study, the position and extent of macroscopic cartilage degeneration and of bone exposure was drawn on an en face map of the patellar surface (Fig. 1.2). A transverse slab was then cut from the patella in the vicinity of the transverse ridge, and photographed to show the articular cartilage and underlying bone in vertical section (Fig. 1.3). The topographical distribution of the lesions was analyzed in terms of lateral, central, and medial patellar segments demarcated as shown in Figure 1.2.

We have found it advisable to analyze the data 1) separately for each age group (since elder patellae may otherwise be over-represented in a necropsy series), and, for some purposes, 2) separately for each sex (since men and women differ in suscep-tibility to patellofemoral osteoarthritis). Several previously pub-lished studies have not taken full account of these factors: any differences between their conclusions and ours can probably be attributed to differences in methods of data analysis, rather than to any basic disagreement about the observations. Further con-fusion arises because there is no uniform nomenclature for anatomical sites on the patellar surface (we ourselves have been inconsistent in our terminology).

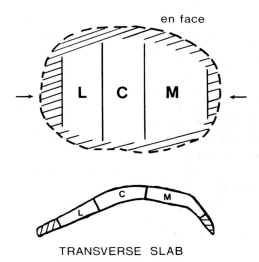

**Figure 1.2.** Diagram of patella en face and in a transverse slab, showing the nomenclature used in the Liverpool study of macroscopically apparent articular cartilage lesions at necropsy: lateral (*L*), central (*C*), and medial (*M*) segments. The transverse slab was cut across the specimens in the vicinity of the transverse ridge (see Figs. 1.3–1.6).

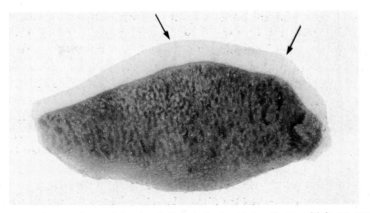

**Figure 1.3.**  Transverse slab of a left patella (unstained) on which no cartilage lesion was macroscopically apparent. The subject was a woman aged 18 years. The lateral facet is on the left of the photograph. Note the contour change of the surface (*arrows*) at the junction between the lateral and main medial facets, and at the junction between the main medial and odd (medial medial) facets.

None of the left patellae from 12 subjects aged 18 to 34 years showed cartilage degeneration sufficiently severe to be apparent on naked eye examination unaided by ink staining of the surface (Fig. 1.3). Macroscopic lesions (Fig. 1.4) were, however, apparent in 12 of 28 subjects aged 35 to 60 years, in 24 of 30 subjects aged 61 to 74 years, and in 17 of 18 subjects aged 75 to 96 years. In some of the subjects, the lesions had become extensive, affecting all three segments of the surface (Fig. 1.5).

In specimens where the macroscopic cartilage degeneration was not too extensive for topographical localization, the lesion was in the vicinity of the transverse ridge. It was localized on the medial or central or both segments in 26 instances, and on the lateral segment in only 2 instances. It will be noted that the central segment includes the junction between the lateral and the main medial patellar facet, and that this junction showed an angled contour of the articular surface when viewed in the vertical slab (Fig. 1.3). The medial segment, as defined for the purpose of our study, included the junction between the main medial facet and the so-called "odd facet" ("most medial facet", "medial area of medial facet"). This junction often also showed an angled contour when viewed in the vertical slab (Figs. 1.3 and 1.4). However, such a medial contour change was absent or

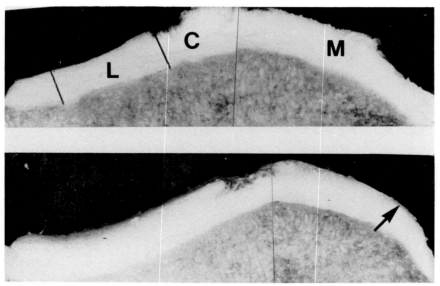

**Figure 1.4.** Transverse slabs from two necropsy specimens of left patellae. In the upper specimen, from a man aged 69 years, lesions macroscopically apparent without ink staining were found on the *C* and also on the *M* segment. In the lower specimen, from a man aged 53 years, a macroscopic lesion was found on the central segment. Note the angled junction (*arrow*) between the main medial and the odd facet. The photographs are of pairs of Polaroid prints and the fine black lines are from the joins.

slight in 14 of 42 left patellae suitable for examination for this anatomical feature.

## ARE THE LESIONS RELATED TO CLINICAL CHONDROMALACIA?

It is of interest to compare the site and age of onset of the macroscopic lesions of patellar cartilage found at necropsy with those reported in patients with clinical "chondromalacia patellae" (patellofemoral pain syndrome). Some of the patients with the clinical syndrome have a macroscopic lesion of their patellar cartilage (5); some have a localized palpable softening of the cartilage without any obvious break in surface continuity (4); the rest have no lesion palpable, or visible on naked eye examination unaided by ink staining. When a lesion is found, it is usually on the medial or central or both segments (2, 4), in the vicinity of the transverse ridge, and often affects the junction

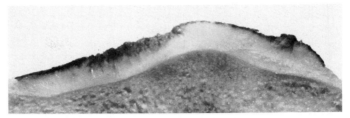

**Figure 1.5.** Extensive involvement of left patellar cartilage by fibrillation which was macroscopically apparent without ink staining. The lateral facet is on the left of the picture. Transverse slab from a patella which had been painted with Indian ink to facilitate photography. Necropsy specimen, woman aged 79 years.

between the main medial and the odd facet, or that between the main medial and the lateral facet. Its topographical distribution thus corresponds to the usual initial sites of the age-related macroscopic cartilage degeneration noted at necropsy in our study. However, in the patellofemoral pain syndrome, the lesions may develop at an age which is earlier than is usual. Thus, Leslie and Bentley (5) found a macroscopic lesion of the patellar cartilage in 11 of 20 patients (55%) aged 20 to 29 years with the patellofemoral pain syndrome, whereas in our study, none of 12 left patellae from necropsy subjects aged 18 to 34 years showed a degenerative change of this severity. It should, however, be noted that formalin fixation of the necropsy cartilages had vitiated examination for any lesions which were palpable but not visible (4).

If the macroscopic lesions seen on the cartilage of some patients with the patellofemoral pain syndrome are of clinical significance, how is it possible that they give rise to symptoms, since cartilage has no nerve endings in it? Are the lesions of no significance at all? Are they in some way responsible for pain coming from the underlying bone? Are they in some way responsible for pain coming from synovial or capsular tissues?

## PATELLOFEMORAL OSTEOARTHRITIS IN NECROPSY MATERIAL

In some older persons, after the age of 50 years, the patellar cartilage degeneration found at necropsy had progressed to bone exposure and bone wear. The appearances were morphologically indistinguishable (Fig. 1.6) from those in surgical excision spec-

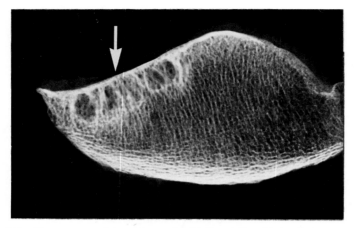

**Figure 1.6.** Transverse slab radiograph of left patella obtained at necropsy from a woman aged 69 years. On the lateral facet (*left of picture*), subarticular bone remodelling, with osteolytic foci interspersed among some osteosclerosis, underlies a destructive cartilage lesion which had progressed to bone exposure (*arrow*).

imens from patients with clinical patellofemoral osteoarthritis. However, the frequency with which the osteoarthritic necropsy lesions were associated with clinical symptoms during life is not known.

Our studies of patellofemoral osteoarthritis in necropsy material led to the following conclusions.

1. The initial site of progression to bone exposure on the patella is usually lateral or central, whereas the initial site of macroscopically apparent cartilage degeneration is usually medial or central (Fig. 1.7). Thus, macroscopic lesions on the lateral and central segments have a greater potential to progress to osteoarthritic bone exposure and bone wear than do lesions on the medial segment (3). This contrast may be related to topographical variation in mechanical stress on patellar cartilage, or to topographical variation in patellar subarticular calcified tissue density (11). The local biomechanical environment of a cartilage lesion, therefore, may affect its natural history.

2. Osteoarthritic patellofemoral bone exposure is more common in older women than in age-matched older men. Possible explanations for a sex difference in osteoarthritis, and the implications of this difference when interpreting laboratory data in cartilage research, have been discussed elsewhere (10).

INITIAL SITES (UNSTAINED PATELLAE)

MACROSCOPIC CARTILAGE LESIONS

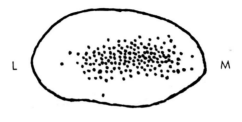

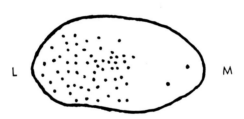

BONE EXPOSURE

**Figure 1.7.**   Diagram showing the distribution of sites at which age-related cartilage degeneration (*top*) first becomes macroscopically apparent on unstained left
patellae at necropsy, compared with the distribution of sites at which age-related
patellar bone exposure (*bottom*) first develops. It should be noted that in the patellar
maps used for this figure the articular surface is intentionally drawn as if it were
laid completely flat, and not angled at the junctions between facets: thus, it is
broader than as drawn in Figure 1.2 and in the "foreshortened" maps of some
other published studies.

 3.  The frequency and severity of patello-femoral osteoarthritis
at necropsy varies between persons of the same age and sex.
 4.  Patellofemoral bone exposure at necropsy often occurs independently of tibiofemoral bone exposure.

## REPAIR OF PATELLAR ARTICULAR CARTILAGE

 When discussing the healing of articular cartilage, it is helpful
to distinguish between two different potential sources of repair:

intrinsic and extrinsic. Intrinsic repair is dependent on the activity of any chondrocytes still surviving at the site of a degenerative lesion. Such cells can multiply and manufacture new matrix, but appear to have difficulty in restoring the continuity of the matrix collagen fiber framework (12). Thus, intrinsic repair has only a limited chance of being effective. Extrinsic repair, in contrast, comes about when new tissue of subarticular origin gains access to the joint surface through gaps in the subarticular bone plate. Such gaps can form as a feature of osteoarthritic change, or can be produced surgically by drilling the bone. The new tissue may spread to re-cover damaged joint surface, and, if chondroid in texture, thus effect a form of cartilaginous repair (12).

### References

1. Bennett GA, Waine H, Bauer W: *Changes in the Knee Joint at Various Ages with Particular Reference to the Nature and Development of Degenerative Joint Disease.* New York, Commonwealth Fund, London, Oxford University Press, 1942.
2. Bentley G, Leslie IJ, Fischer D: Effect of aspirin treatment on chondromalacia patellae. *Ann Rheum Dis* 40:37–41, 1981.
3. Emery IH, Meachim G: Surface morphology and topography of patello-femoral cartilage fibrillation in Liverpool necropsies. *J Anat* 116:103–120, 1973.
4. Goodfellow J, Hungerford DS, Woods C: Patello-femoral joint mechanics and pathology. 2: Chondromalacia Patellae. *J Bone Joint Surg* 58-B:291–299, 1976.
5. Leslie IJ, Bentley G: Arthroscopy in the diagnosis of chondromalacia patellae. *Ann Rheum Dis* 37:540–547, 1978.
6. Meachim G: Effect of age on the thickness of adult articular cartilage at the shoulder joint. *Ann Rheum Dis* 30:43–46, 1971.
7. Meachim G, Bentley G: Horizontal splitting in patellar articular cartilage. *Arthritis Rheum* 21:669–674, 1978.
8. Meachim G, Bentley G, Baker R: Effect of age on thickness of adult patellar cartilage. *Ann Rheum Dis* 36:563–568, 1977.
9. Meachim G, Denham D, Emery IH, et al: Collagen alignments and artificial splits at the surface of human articular cartilage. *J Anat* 118:101–118, 1974.
10. Meachim G, Pedley RB: Implications of a sex difference in osteoarthrosis. *Ann Rheum Dis* 39:199, 1980.
11. Pedley, RB, Meachim G: Topographical variation in patellar subarticular calcified tissue density. *J Anat* 128:737–745, 1979.
12. Stockwell RA, Meachim G: The Chondrocytes. In Freeman MAR: *Adult Articular Cartilage*, 2nd edition. London, Pitman, 1979, pp 69–144.

CHAPTER TWO

# Patellar Position, Patellar Osteotomy—Their Relationship to Chondromalacia: X-Ray Diagnosis of Chondromalacia

CARROLL LAURIN, M.D.

There are many potential causes of chondromalacia as elaborated in an etiological classification (Table 2.1). I wish to discuss the mechanical pathogenesis of chondromalacia. I shall elaborate on the x-ray diagnosis of chondromalacia by attempting to answer three questions:

1. Can experimental patellar malalignment induce chondromalacia patellae?

2. Can patellar malalignment be quantitated radiologically?

3. Is it, in fact, possible to diagnose chondromalacia patellae radiologically?

## EXPERIMENTAL INDUCTION OF CHONDROMALACIA

We attempted to induce patellar malalignment in dogs by doing an anteriorly based sagittal wedge resection of the patella, combined with a medial capsulotomy, to tilt the patella, and thus, possibly defunction the medial patellofemoral joint. On the control side, we performed a sagittal osteotomy, a medial capsulotomy but no wedge resection of bone was removed from the patella. As expected, we encountered many technical difficulties with patellar osteotomies, most of them related to the fact that the patella in dogs is hard, round, small, thus making the osteotomy and the osteosynthesis very difficult. In the few animals where osteosynthesis was maintained, we did achieve

11

**Table 2.1.**
**Classification of Chondromalacia Patella (Etiology)**

1. Mechanical
2. Inflammatory
3. Degenerative
4. Post-traumatic
5. Dystrophic
6. Vascular
7. Idiopathic

defunctioning of the medial patellofemoral compartment and medial malacic lesions. However, these lesions were bilateral making their interpretation difficult in terms of the responsible pathogenesis.

The experiment, therefore, was modified on the control side and no patellar osteotomy was performed; rather, the medial capsulotomy was left unrepaired. The procedure was unchanged on the experimental side in 23 animals.

Somewhat to our surprise, both procedures, on the experimental and control sides, achieved defunctioning of the medial patellofemoral joint with malacic lesions on both sides of the medial patellofemoral compartment, namely, the patellar and femoral sides.

Since the medial capsulotomy appeared to be sufficient to induce malacic lesions, as performed on the control side, the experiment, therefore, was modified one more time; an unrepaired capsulotomy was performed on the experimental side while the capsulotomy was repaired on the control side.

Malacic lesions of the medial compartment of the patellofemoral joint were noted on the experimental side only and again on both sides of the medial patellofemoral joint. These lesions were graded histologically by noting the uptake of safarin O, the presence or absence of horizontal and vertical fissuring, and finally, the incidence of cloning. Indeed the histology of the experimental lesions closely resembled the histology noted in clinical chondromalacia.

In conclusion, it was possible to achieve patellar malalignment by three experiments, the simplest being an unrepaired medial capsulotomy. All seemed to achieve patellar malalignment and experimental malacic lesions which macroscopically and microscopically corresponded to chondromalacia and we could state that patellar malalignment, at least in dogs, can induce patellofemoral chondromalacia experimentally.

The next pertinent question that must be considered is whether patellar malalignment indeed can be quantitated radiologically.

There are, of course, different types of patellar malalignment: namely, up or down, side to side, dynamic, or static.

We shall only consider static, side to side patellar malalignment, as assessed on the axial x-ray of the patellofemoral joint. If we wish to quantitate this x-ray image, it becomes obvious that the x-ray technique must be standardized, first by rigidly controlling three variables as well as by elaborating a reliable mode of objective assessment of the x-ray image.

The first variable to control is the position of the patient who may be prone, seated, kneeling, or supine.

In the prone position, the knees may be in a position of hyperflexion or semiextension; in the flexed position, as we shall see later, we then are visualizing the wrong segment, namely, the distal or tibial segment of the patellofemoral groove. When the knees are in a position of almost complete extension or mild flexion, the x-ray plate is then necessarily at 45° to the x-ray tube with inevitable distortion of the x-ray image making the measurement or quantitative assessment of the x-ray image difficult. If the patient is kneeling on the x-ray plate, we then have the worst of both worlds, namely, the knee is in a position of hyperflexion while the x-ray plate is at 45° to the x-ray tube with distortion of the x-ray image. We may conclude then that the patient must be supine or seated (6).

The second variable to control is obviously the position of the knee. Most authors would now agree that we must, at all cost, avoid the former skyline view, during which the knees are in a position of hyperflexion; the reason is that then we are visualizing the wrong segment of the patellofemoral joint, since we are looking at the tibial segment. It is now well recognized that the patella is unstable at the proximal segment of the femoral groove and this is the segment that must be visualized radiologically as beautifully demonstrated in sequential tangential x-rays where the patellar tilt will be seen to be obvious with the knees in a position of 20–30° of flexion while the diagnosis is completely missed, with a false, normal image, with the knees flexed at 40° or 50° (1).

While other techniques have their relative advantages, we believe that the best method is the one whereby the patient is supine, the knees at rest on a support, 20° short of complete extension (Fig. 2.1A).

Finally, the x-ray technique, or the relationship between the x-ray plate, the x-ray tube, and the knees must be standardized. As in the x-ray visualization of any joint, an optimal image will be obtained if x-rays are parallel to the joint and at 90° to the plate. To respect these requirements when visualizing the patellofemoral joint axially, the x-ray beam should be parallel to the anterior border of the tibia while the plate is held proximally by the patient, at 90° to the x-ray beam (2, 4) (Fig. 2.1B).

Using this x-ray technique, the patellofemoral joint should appear at the bottom of the x-ray plate (Fig. 2.1C); occasionally, particularly in obese patients, the patellofemoral joint is too low and may not be well visualized. It is very important to repeat the x-ray exposure in the following manner: the position of the x-ray tube must not be changed, the knees must not be flexed further; rather, the x-ray plate should be moved proximally as the patient pushes downward on the quadriceps. Should the knees have been flexed by mistake, the wrong segment of the patellofemoral joint will be visualized; should the x-ray plate have been laid flat against the femur, you get obvious distortion of the patella since the plate is then at 45° to the x-ray beam. This opportunity to adjust the position of the plate manually is a distinct advantage of this technique (3, 4).

---

**Figure 2.1.** *A.* X-ray technique: The knee is in the 160° position (20° short of complete extension). The x-ray source is usually below the table top and directed in the cephalad direction; the x-rays are parallel to the anterior border of the tibia and to the patellofemoral interspace; the x-ray plate is at 90° to the x-rays and to the patellofemoral interspace. *B.* The x-rays are parallel to the patellofemoral joint when the knee is positioned in the 160° position and the x-ray plate should be at 90° to the beam and to the patellofemoral joint. *C.* Characteristic image of the patellofemoral interspace when the x-ray technique is performed as described: the x-ray image of the patella corresponds to a crosssection of that same patella; the lateral patellofemoral compartment is wider; the lateral femoral condyle is rounded, while the medial femoral condyle has a sharp contour (*arrow*). Reprinted with permission from Laurin et al., *Clin Orthop* 144:16–18, 1979 (4).

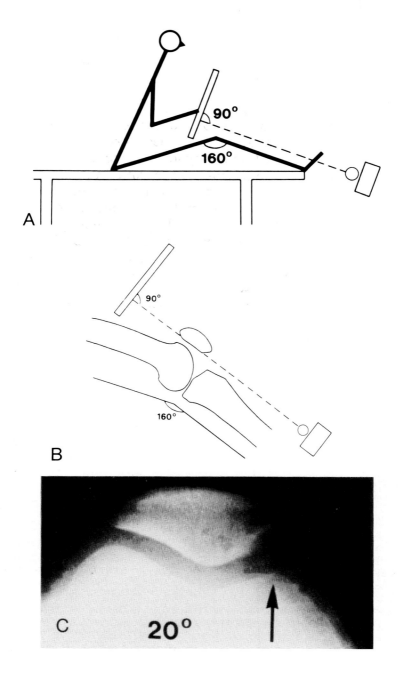

Once the x-ray technique had been standardized, it was logical to wish to quantitate the x-ray image. In the past, we tended merely to eyeball the patellofemoral joint. Without any objective measurement of the image as illustrated in patients where malalignment may seem to be obvious on one side only but not so obvious on the opposite side although we are, in fact, dealing with bilateral lesions. Patellar position can be assessed by drawing lines on the axial x-ray image to assess the patellofemoral index (P.F.I), the lateral patellar displacement, and the lateral patellofemoral angle (P.F.A.) (5).

The patellofemoral angle is designed to quantitate patellar tilt, it can be calculated by drawing two lines: one joining the anterior borders of the femoral condyles and another line joining the limits of the lateral patellar facet (Fig. 2.2A). The reason for choosing the limits of the lateral patellar facet, as reference points of the patella, is that the shape of the medial facet changes, while the contour of the lateral patellar facet is constant, an anatomical observation which is the basis of the Wiberg classification of patellar shapes. The normal patellofemoral angle is open laterally; as the patella tilts, the lines are first parallel and, eventually, the patellofemoral angle will be reversed (Fig. 2.2B).

We also wished to assess lateral patellar displacement objectively. To do so, a vertical line is drawn at 90° to line A at the anterior edge of the medial femoral condyle (5) (Figs. 2.1 and 2.3).

The third objective sign that we looked for was the actual shape of the patella to determine whether, in fact, different shapes of the patella were associated with different patellar syndromes (7).

While the patellofemoral angle would allow us to detect major tilts of the patella, it seemed that we needed a more sensitive x-ray sign to detect minitilts of the patella or mild patellar malalignment, if indeed such a thing existed. To do so, we proposed the patellofemoral index which is merely a ratio comparing the thicknesses of the medial and lateral patellar joint spaces (4). By using a standardized x-ray technique and by referring to four objective criteria, it was possible to quantitate patellar malalignment radiologically.

We were ready now to consider the third question, namely: "is it possible to diagnose chondromalacia patellae radiologi-

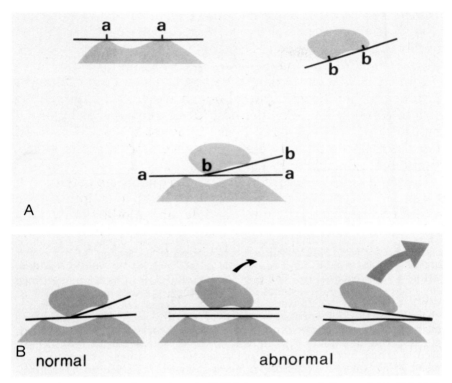

**Figure 2.2.** *A.* Patellofemoral angle (P.F.A.) measurement: line aa joins the summits of the femoral condyles, line bb joins the limits of the lateral patellar facette, and the patellofemoral angle is situated above line aa, where it is crossed by line bb. *B.* Normal and abnormal patellofemoral angles. The normal patellofemoral angle is always open laterally; there is no need to measure the angle since it varies considerably from one individual to the other and also with the same individual, if the x-rays are taken at different degrees of knee flexion or extension. It is vital, therefore, that the technique be standardized with x-rays taken at the 20° position. As the patella tilts laterally, the lines become parallel in 40% of patients with recurrent dislocation of the patella (R.D.P.); as the patella tilts further, the patellofemoral angle is reversed and is now open medially. The degree of tilt of the patella in chondromalacia is not sufficient to modify the patellofemoral angle sufficiently to render the two lines parallel or to reverse the patellofemoral angle. For that reason, the patellofemoral angle is not proposed to recognize chondromalacia patellae radiologically.

cally?" At this point, we made two assumptions: one, that experimentally and clinically, there appeared to be a relevant relationship between patellar malalignment and chondromalacia patellae (2). The second presumption was that there are

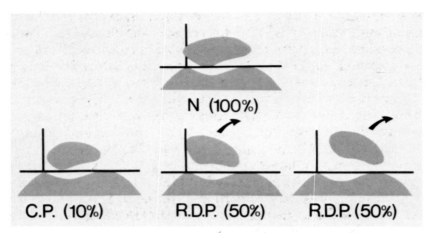

**Figure 2.3.**   Lateral patellar displacement. Lateral patellar displacement can be assessed objectively by drawing a line perpendicular to line aa, at the medial femoral condyle. In normal individuals, the patella touches the vertical line or is medial to it. In recurrent dislocation of the patella (R.D.P.), the tilt is associated with a lateral shift in 50% of cases (*right lower drawing*) while in 50% of patients there is a tilt of the patella without any lateral displacement. In chondromalacia patellae, there is a lateral shift of the patella in only 10% of patients. Hence, lateral patellar displacement is not considered a reliable x-ray sign of chondromalacia patellae. There is possibly a better way to assess lateral patellar displacement which is almost inevitably seen in patellofemoral osteoarthritis; conceivably, in those patients where the patellofemoral osteoarthritis was preceded by chondromalacia patellae, lateral patellar displacement should or could nave been detected before the onset of patellofemoral osteoarthritis. The proposed method of measurement of lateral patellar displacement, therefore, is possibly not sufficient.

different degrees of patellar malalignment: severe malalignment leads to recurrent dislocation of the patella (R.D.P.) while mild patellar malalignment would be associated with chondromalacia (C.P.). The logical extension of these two assumptions is that patellar malalignment must be quantitated radiologically if we wished to diagnose chondromalacia patellae radiologically (3, 4).

A control population of 100 normal patients was compared with 100 patients suffering from chondromalacia and with 30 patients with recurrent dislocation of the patella. The clinical diagnoses were made by a surgeon who was not involved with the interpretation of the x-ray images.

It became obvious that the patellofemoral angle was a reliable sign to assess the degree of patellar tilt objectively. Although the angle varied in normal individuals, the lateral patellofemoral angle was almost always open laterally, namely, in 97% of normal individuals; while 3% of normal candidates had abnormal, parallel lines, none of the normal individuals had a reverse patellofemoral angle (Fig. 2.4). In recurrent dislocation of the patella, however, reversal of the patellofemoral angle is noted in 40% of patients while 60% had parallel lines. This observation is only valid if the x-ray technique is such that the knees are x-rayed in the 20° position; it should be noted that the angle resumes to normal if the knees are flexed (Table 2.2).

The lateral patellofemoral angle, however, was grossly inadequate to diagnose chondromalacia patellae and was abnormal and parallel in only 10% of patients with chondromalacia, very likely because the degree of tilt was not severe enough to reverse the patellofemoral angle (Fig. 2.4).

The incidence of lateral patellar displacement also was disappointing as an x-ray sign to diagnose chondromalacia radiologically. While 50% of patients with a dislocating patella had excessive lateral displacement, only 10% of patients with chondromalacia exhibited significant lateral patellar displacement (Fig. 2.3).

The patellofemoral index (Fig. 2.5), a ratio comparing the medial and lateral compartment thicknesses, depends on an accurate assessment of both compartments as well as on a standardized x-ray technique. The assessment or measurement of the lateral compartment, as indicated by L, is relatively easy; on the medial side, this measurement is complicated by the changing shape of the medial facet. Hence, the landmark on the patella corresponds to the actual junction between the lateral and medial facets of the patella. The femoral landmark to assess

**Table 2.2.**
**X-Ray Signs (in the 20° Position)**

| | Lateral P.F.A. | | | Patellar Displacement | | P.F.I. | |
|---|---|---|---|---|---|---|---|
| | Open Laterally | Parallel | Open Medially | Medial to or Touching Line "C" | Lateral to Line "C" | 1.0 or Less | More than 1.0 |
| Normal controls | 97% | 3% | 0% | 100% | 0% | 100% | 0% |
| Subluxing patellae | 0% | 60% | 40% | 47% | 53% | 0% | 100% |
| Chondromalacia patellae | 90% | 10% | 0% | 70% | 30% | 3% | 97% |

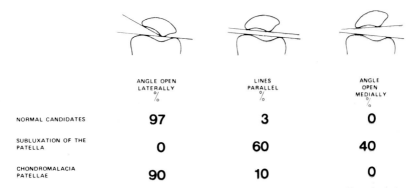

| | ANGLE OPEN LATERALLY % | LINES PARALLEL % | ANGLE OPEN MEDIALLY % |
|---|---|---|---|
| NORMAL CANDIDATES | 97 | 3 | 0 |
| SUBLUXATION OF THE PATELLA | 0 | 60 | 40 |
| CHONDROMALACIA PATELLAE | 90 | 10 | 0 |

**Figure 2.4.** Patellofemoral angle in three population groups. Reprinted with permission from Laurin et al., *Clin Orthop* 144:25, 1979 (4).

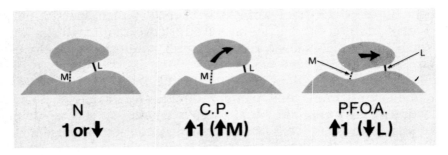

**Figure 2.5.** The patellofemoral index (M/L). This index is the relationship between the relative thickness of the medial patellofemoral compartment (*M*) and the lateral patello-femoral compartment (*L*). Measurement *L* corresponds to the shortest distance between the lateral patellar facette and the lateral femoral condyle. Measurement *M* is the shortest distance between the medial femoral groove and the junction between the medial and lateral patellar facettes. The junction between the medial and lateral patellar facettes corresponds to the lateral edge of the patellar facette and is proposed as a point of reference, since it is the only constant point on the medial patellar facette whose shape changes from one individual to the other (and, thus, is the basis of the Wiberg classification) and also changes in the same individual if one visualizes different segments of the medial patellar facette. In normal individuals, the *M* over *L* relationship, the patellofemoral index, is 1 or less; occasionally measurement *L* is larger than measurement *M* but, in normal individuals, measurement *M* is never larger than measurement *L* when tangential views are taken in the recommended technique. The patellofemoral index is abnormal, i.e., greater than 1 in chondromalacia patellae because measurement *M* is increased, and, in lateral patellofemoral osteoarthritis because measurement *L* is decreased.

the thickness of the medial patellofemoral joint corresponds to the shortest distance between the patellar reference point and the closest segment of the medial femoral groove. In normal individuals, this patellofemoral ratio or patellofemoral index (M/L) measures 1 or less, since the lateral patellofemoral joint is sometimes larger but is never smaller than the medial patellofemoral joint space (4) (Fig. 2.5).

In chondromalacia patients, there is a gentle tilt of the patella increasing measurement M; hence, in chondromalacia, the patellofemoral index (M/L) is larger than 1. Using this measurement, the patellofemoral index, it was possible to diagnose chondromalacia in 93% of patients in this series as the patellofemoral index was then larger than 1.

It is interesting to note that in lateral patellofemoral osteoarthritis, as measurement L decreases, the patellofemoral index (M/L) also increases (4) (Fig. 2.5).

In cases of recurrent dislocation of the patella, since we then are dealing with a more important tilt of the patella, as made obvious by a reverse patellofemoral angle, the patellofemoral index (M/L) is always abnormal and measures more than 1 as measurement M, or the medial patellofemoral compartment distance, far exceeds measurement L.

The patellofemoral index in normal individuals, thus, is one or less; for different reasons, the patellofemoral index is more than 1 in chondromalacia and in patellofemoral osteoarthritis. In chondromalacia patellae, the patellofemoral index is more than 1 because measurement M has increased while in patellofemoral osteoarthritis, patellofemoral index is again larger than 1 but because measurement L has decreased (Fig. 2.5). The patellofemoral angle, therefore, is a good and reliable x-ray sign for gross patellar tilt as shown in recurrent dislocation of the patella. The patellofemoral index is a reliable x-ray sign of minitilt of the patella, namely, chondromalacia where the patellofemoral angle may be normal while the patellofemoral index is abnormal and greater than 1 (Fig. 2.6 and Table 2.2).

The incidence of different patellar contours was also calculated for the three population groups. Wiberg types 1, 2, and 3 were distributed randomly in the three population groups (7); however, the Bomgardtl type 4 patella, or the unifacet patella,

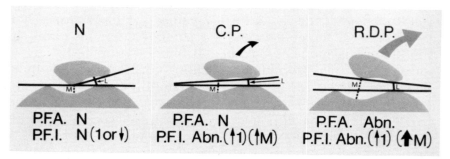

**Figure 2.6.**  Relationship between patellofemoral angle (P.F.A.) and the patello-femoral index (P.F.I.). Both measurements (P.F.A. and P.F.I.) are objective methods of measuring patellar tilt. The patellofemoral angle is easier to draw and will pick up more obvious types of patellar tilt, as seen in recurrent dislocation of the patella. The patellofemoral index is more difficult to draw but is an accurate method of objectively assessing and recognizing a minitilt of the patella as seen in chondro-malacia. Hence, in normal individuals, the patellofemoral angle is normal and open laterally, while the patellofemoral index is equally normal and measures 1 or less. In recurrent dislocation of the patella, the patellofemoral angle is an easier method of assessing this obvious patellar tilt; since the patellofemoral index is a more sensitive method of measuring patellar tilt it is also abnormal. Since the patello-femoral index is possibly more difficult to draw and interpret, it is usually easier to make the diagnosis of recurrent dislocation of the patella by referring to the patellofemoral angle which is always abnormal (in 40% of cases the patellofemoral angle is reversed and open medially while in 60% of cases the lines are parallel). In chondromalacia, the tilt of the patella is not sufficient to render the patellofemoral angle abnormal although it is decreased and less than is usually seen in normal candidates; hence, this method of assessing the x-ray image is not proposed to recognize chondromalacia. The patellofemoral index, however, is more critical and more sensitive and will pick up a minitilt of the patella as seen in 93% of patients with chondromalacia.

was never seen in normal individuals but was seen in patients with chondromalacia or recurrent dislocation of the patella. The unifacet patella is not a frequent contour but, when seen, it should suggest chondromalacia or recurrent dislocation of the patella.

Finally, a word of caution is indicated since patellar malalign-ment may not always be radiologically obvious in patients with clinically proven chondromalacia. There are three possible ex-planations: the first and likeliest, is that the x-ray protocol was not respected; second, the patellar malalignment may be very mild or it may be the vertical, "up and down" type of patellar malalignment; and finally, we may be dealing with a nonme-chanical cause of chondromalacia.

In conclusion, we can answer our three original questions:

1. Yes, it is possible to induce chondromalacia in dogs by experimental malalignment.

2. Yes, we can assess patellar malalignment radiologically as long as a rigid x-ray protocol is respected with the x-ray tube parallel to the anterior border of the tibia, the x-ray plate at 90° to the patellofemoral joint, and the knees, at rest in a 20° position.

3. And finally, yes, it is possible to diagnose chondromalacia radiologically and the following signs are of assistance: the patellar shape, the patellofemoral angle, and patellofemoral index.

### References

1. Ficat RP, Hungerford DS: *Disorders of the Patello-Femoral Joint.* Baltimore, The Williams & Wilkins Co, 1977.
2. Hughston JC: Subluxation of the Patella. *J Bone Joint Surg* 50-A:1003–1026, 1968.
3. Labelle H, Peides JP, Levesque HP, et al: Evaluation de la position rotulienne en incidence radiographique tangentielle. *Union Med Con* 105:870, 1976.
4. Laurin CA, Dussault R, Levesque HP: The tangential x-ray investigation of the patellofemoral joint. X-ray technique, diagnostic criteria and their interpretation. *Clin Orthop* 144:16–26, 1979.
5. Laurin CA, Levesque HP, Dussault R, et al: The abnormal lateral patello-femoral angle. A diagnostic, roentgenographic sign of recurrent subluxation. *J Bone Joint Surg* 60-A:55–60, 1978.
6. Merchant AC, Mercer RL, Jacobson RH, et al: Roentgenographic analysis of patello-femoral congruence. *J Bone Joint Surg* 56-A:1391–1396, 1974.
7. Wiberg G: Roentgenographic and anatomic studies of the femoro-patellar joint. *Acta Orthop Scand* 12:319–410, 1941.

# CHAPTER THREE

# Patellar Subluxation and Excessive Lateral Pressure as a Cause of Fibrillation

**DAVID S. HUNGERFORD, M.D.**

I have been asked to discuss the relationship between patellar subluxation, the excessive lateral pressure syndrome (ELPS) and articular cartilage fibrillation of the patella. However, this presupposes that the definition of articular cartilage fibrillation is universally understood and that there is some determinable relationship between fibrillation and the subject of this symposium, chondromalacia patellae. Since both of these suppositions are subjects of considerable controversy, my remarks can only be understood in the context of my own prejudices.

## THE TERM "CHONDROMALACIA PATELLAE"

Although the term chondromalacia patellae is commonly used as a synonym for patellofemoral arthralgia, arthritis, or even anterior knee pain, it is not useful to do so. Chondromalacia patellae is simply a multifaceted disorder of the articular cartilage on the undersurface of the patellae in which the articular cartilage is softened and fibrillated. This may or may not be associated with symptoms which, in and of itself, pose a large practical clinical problem. With arthroscopy, it is easy to identify malacic lesions of patellar articular cartilage, but are the patient's symptoms the results of the lesion?

It is perhaps useful to examine how we have arrived at the current state of affairs whereby this term, chondromalacia patellae, has lost its specificity and usefulness. Prior to 1936, the term "chondromalacia patellae post-traumatica" was useful and specific. It was coined by Aleman (1) and widely used in Scandinavia to depict a lesion on the undersurface of the patella, as a result of trauma, associated with symptoms, and discovered at arthrotomy. However, the publication of Owre's pathological

24

study in 1936 (14), followed by Hirsch in 1941 (9), used the same term without the "traumatica" to describe a lesion in cadavers in which an association with trauma or symptoms could not be determined.

Then, beginning in the late 1940s, we started to get clinical descriptions of patellofemoral pain syndromes in which the term chondromalacia patellae was used (2, 3, 5, 13). Next, a paper was published on the bony changes of "chondromalacia patellae" in which 13 of 17 specimens showed no lesions of articular cartilage (4). More recently, some clinical papers have appeared in which the articular cartilage itself was not even evaluated, even though the authors were allegedly defining the characteristics of chondromalacia patellae (15).

I would submit that chondromalacia patellae as a term is the equivalent in usefulness for the orthopaedist as the nephrotic syndrome is for the nephrologist. That is, the nephrotic syndrome means the kidney does not work very well and chondromalacia patellae means that the cartilage is abnormal, nothing more. Therefore, when chondromalacia is encountered, relationship to symptoms and possible etiological relationships must be determined. It must be clearly remembered, when you have said chondromalacia patellae, you have said virtually nothing of any practical usefulness, you have definitely not "said it all."

## FIBRILLATION

There remains one more problem to resolve before launching into the main topic. All fibrillation is not equal. Surface fibrillation affects those areas of articular cartilage which are either out of contact with other articular surfaces or are habitual noncontact areas, i.e., during most activity they are not in contact. The cumbersome but descriptively accurate term of nonprogressive, age-dependent surface fibrillation has been coined for these lesions which usually involve only the C-1 layer of articular cartilage (8). There is no indication that these lesions are ever associated with symptoms. They are, however, important to recognize so as not to misinterpret their significance when they are encountered at surgery or arthroscopy.

The second kind of cartilage lesion on the patella involves the weight-bearing zone, and corresponds to those areas which demonstrate full-thickness cartilage loss in cases of patello-femoral arthritis. It is difficult to determine the rate of progression of these cartilage lesions to cartilage loss but they certainly occur in the same area. This cartilage lesion is best referred to as fasciculation rather than fibrillation because the pattern is coarser, and the lesion invariably extends into the deep layers of articular cartilage (Fig. 3.1).

Occasionally, the earliest form of this lesion may be encountered as a blister on the articular surface (Fig. 3.2) in which the surface appears to be macroscopically intact. In this blister lesion, the deeper layers are disrupted, allowing the proteoglycans to imbibe additional water causing the cartilage swelling, i.e., the swelling of the proteoglycans is no longer constrained by the intact collagen network. Once the lesion breaks through the surface, having begun as a lesion in the deeper layers, it first appears as deep coarse clefts into the depths of the articular cartilage. Paul Ficat and I (7) have schematized the hypothetical progression of this kind of lesion from its earliest appearance through to complete loss of the articular cartilage (Fig. 3.3).

## PATELLOFEMORAL CONTACT AREA

My principal thesis will be to demonstrate that patellofemoral malalignment and instability dramatically alter the contact area

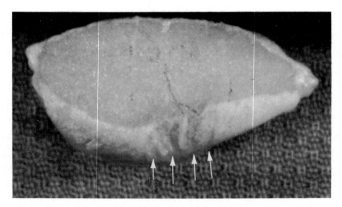

**Figure 3.1.** Cross-section of a patella showing deep coarse fasciculation into the deeper layers of the central zone. Reprinted with permission from Ficat and Hungerford, *Disorders of the Patello-femoral Joint.* Baltimore, Williams & Wilkins, 1977 (7).

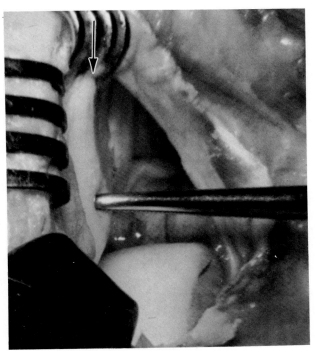

**Figure 3.2.**    Blister lesion with macroscopically intact surface can be abnormally compressed. Reprinted with permission from Ficat and Hungerford, *Disorders of the Patello-femoral Joint.* Baltimore, Williams & Wilkins, 1977 (7).

of the patellofemoral joint, with resultant change in the contact stress. However, first it is appropriate to review the normal contact areas and how force is transferred across the patello-femoral joint. It can be seen from Figure 3.4 that the contact area begins at the inferior surface of the patella as it is drawn into the trochlear groove. It extends as a broad band from the lateral margin of the patella to the ridge separating the medial and the odd facets. As flexion proceeds, that band moves proximally on the patella and distally on the trochlea, but respecting the boundary separating the medial and odd facets (Fig. 3.4B). This band increases in area steadily up to 90° of flexion when the contact area has reached the proximal margin of the patellar articular surface (Fig. 3.4C). It should be noted that throughout this range, from 0–90° flexion, the odd facet has remained out of contact.

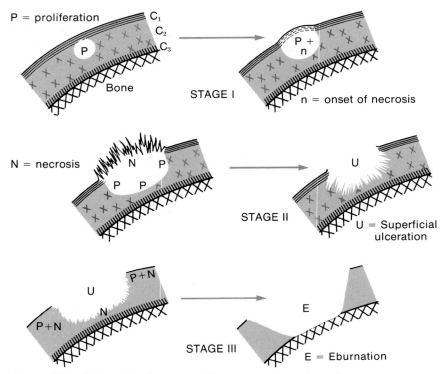

**Figure 3.3.** Schematic diagram of the progression of cartilage lesions of the patella. Reprinted with permission from Ficat and Hungerford, *Disorders of the Patello-femoral Joint.* Baltimore, Williams & Wilkins, 1977 (7).

Beyond 90° flexion, the quadriceps tendon begins to come into high pressure contact with the proximal margin of the trochlea, so that the patellofemoral joint reaction (PFJR) force is transferred across both a patellofemoral contact area and a tendofemoral contact area (Fig. 3.4D, E). Also, the medial contact begins to flow over onto the odd facet. This transition occurs at the proximal margin of the patella where the *ridge* separating the medial and odd facets is minimal or nonexistant, so that in most instances this should be a smooth shift. By 135° of flexion, the medial and lateral contact areas are completely separated with the medial area restricted only to the odd facet and the medial facet out of contact in the intercondylar notch (Fig. 3.4E). The tendofemoral contact zone has increased dramatically in area.

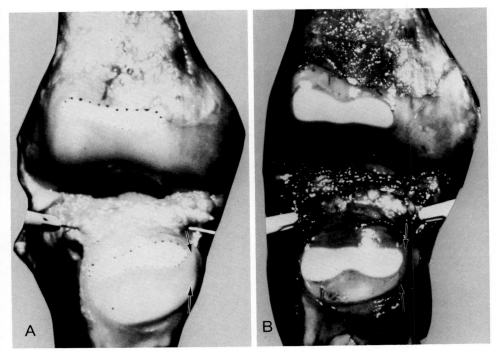

**Figure 3.4.** Normal patellofemoral contact areas for increasing degrees of flexion: A. 20°; B. 60°; C. 90°; D, 120°; E. 135°. Reprinted with permission from Ficat and Hungerford, *Disorders of the Patello-femoral Joint.* Baltimore, Williams & Wilkins, 1977 (7).

This then is the "field of combat", so to speak, over which the PFJR force flows. However, it is useless to talk about contact area in an absence of consideration of the magnitude of the joint reaction force. Too often, the reverse has been true, changes in total force have been calculated or measured without any consideration of possible changes in contact area. In the end analysis, unit load is all that counts. Chondrocytes and collagen fibers are damaged by *unit load* and, from a physical point of view, only unit load.

## BIOMECHANICS OF THE PATELLOFEMORAL JOINT

The complete biomechanics of the patellofemoral joint is beyond the scope of this presentation, and is not even fully worked out in detail. However, broad principles are understood

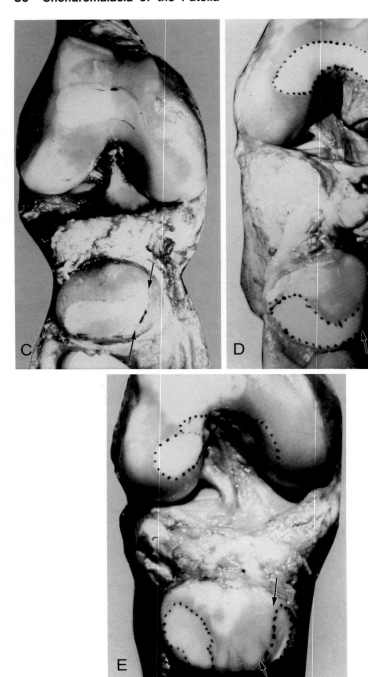

**Figure 3.4.**   C–E.

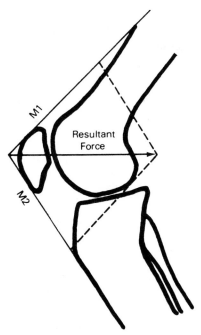

**Figure 3.5.** The PFJR force is that vector of the tension developed in the quadriceps and patellar tendons which is directed against the joint. Redrawn from Ficat and Hungerford, *Disorders of the Patello-femoral Joint.* Baltimore, Williams & Wilkins, 1977 (7).

and applicable to this discussion. The patella is compressed against the trochlea by the tension that develops in the quadriceps and patellar tendons (Fig. 3.5). This tension is developed by the quadriceps muscle in response to bending moments about the knee. When the center of gravity lies in front of the instant center of the knee, there is no force tending to flex the knee and therefore no quadriceps tension is necessary. PFJR force will be zero (Fig. 3.6A).

As the knee is flexed under load, the center of gravity falls increasingly behind the center of rotation of the knee. This increasing flexor lever arm (x in Fig. 3.6B) increases the moment, requiring an increasing response from the quadriceps to balance it. Therefore, with increasing knee flexion, there is an increase in the force of quadriceps contraction. This alone would be sufficient to cause an increase in the PFJR force. However, the *proportion* of quadriceps tension which is translated into patellar

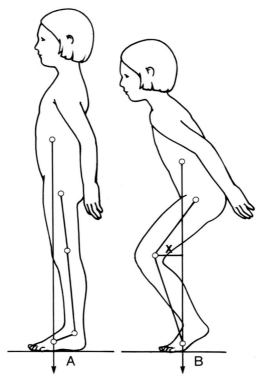

**Figure 3.6.** A. With the center of gravity in front of the knee, no quadriceps force is required. B. As the center of gravity passes behind the instant center of the knee, the flexor lever arm, x, increases with increasing flexion. Reprinted with permission from Ficat and Hungerford, *Disorders of the Patello-femoral Joint.* Baltimore, Williams & Wilkins, 1977 (7).

compression against the trochlea is a function of the angle between the quadriceps tendon and the patellar tendon. When that angle is 180°, as it nearly is in full extension, there is little or no compression of the patella against the femur regardless of the tension which is developed in the quadriceps tendon. As the knee flexes and as the angle between the quadriceps tension and patellar tendon increases, the percentage of quadriceps tension which is directed against the patellofemoral articulation increases as well. Therefore, with increasing knee flexion, *two* factors work together synergistically to increase PFJR force: 1) the increasing flexor lever arm requires an increasing quadriceps response; and 2) the increasing angle between the quadriceps tendon and the patellar tendon directs an increasing percentage of that response toward the patellofemoral joint.

If we then look again at the contact pattern of the patellofemoral joint, we can see that there is an increase in the contact area for dissipating this increase in patellofemoral load with increasing flexion. Although this increase is not sufficient to maintain a constant unit load throughout the range of motion, it is sufficient to reduce the unit load significantly under what it would be if there were no change in contact area throughout the range of flexion. This represents, therefore, a sophisticated and subtle mechanism within the patellofemoral joint, which sees very high loads, for reducing unit load. This is the normal framework within which pathological situations such as subluxation occur.

## EFFECT OF PATELLAR SUBLUXATION ON THE CONTACT AREA

We used the same testing set-up for evaluating the effect of patellar subluxation on the contact area that we used for carrying out the contact studies on the normal joint (Fig. 3.7). The tibia is mounted vertically in the test rig and clamped to the table. Through an intramedullary rod in the femur to which a winch is attached, the quadriceps tendon is fixed with a wire threaded through the substance of the tendon. The position of the joint then is determined by the length of the "quadriceps tendon" which can be varied by shortening or lengthening it through turning the winch. A weight is hung from the intramedullary rod. This system allows complete freedom of rotation of the femur around the vertical axis of the tibia and, therefore, allows the femur to settle into the neutral plane of rotation. Through independent studies, it was demonstrated that active internal rotation of the femur on the fixed tibia would lead to lateral subluxation of the patella, particularly in the first 30° of flexion (10). For the purposes of this study, contact prints were made at 30° of knee flexion and then, using another dye, a second contact print was made with the patella in minimal subluxation which was produced by internally rotating the femur on the fixed tibia. This, in fact, is a very common mechanism for patellar subluxation and dislocation; that is, a turning movement off the fixed foot with the knee in 30° of flexion or

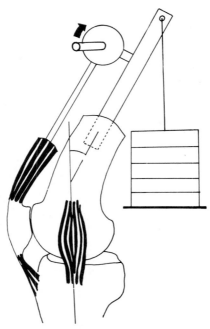

**Figure 3.7.**  Test rig for loading the patellofemoral joint when obtaining contact print. Redrawn from Ficat and Hungerford, *Disorders of the Patello-femoral Joint.* Baltimore, Williams & Wilkins, 1977 (7).

less. The two contact areas are shown superimposed on Figure 3.8. The broad bend of contact at 30° of flexion in the normal state measures 2.24 cm². Minimal subluxation changed the entire pattern of the contact from a broad band extending from the lateral border of the patella to the ridge separating the medial and odd facets to a circular area of contact just lateral to the median ridge, reducing the area of contact to 0.94 cm², a reduction of more than 60%. If PFJR force has not been reduced by this subluxation, and there is no reason to suppose that it would be, this simple change in contact area would increase the contact stress by 2½ times. I do not believe it is mere coincidence that this area superimposes almost perfectly onto the critical zone which Paul Ficat and I have described (Fig. 3.9). This zone was defined by morphological studies on cadaver knees and arthrographic studies of the patellofemoral joint as that area of the articular cartilage which is most often affected by deep fissures,

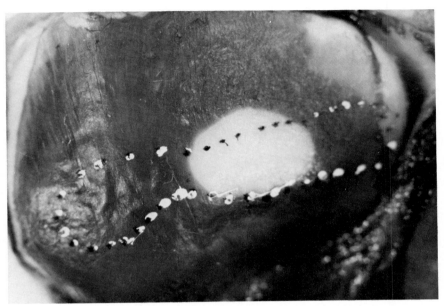

**Figure 3.8.**   Contact prints in 30° of flexion, the broad band. The broad band is the normal contact pattern while the circular area lateral to the median ridge is the pattern with minimal lateral subluxation.

the so-called open lesion of chondromalacia patellae. It would appear that whatever else might be wrong with the patello-femoral joint or whatever procedures might be carried out to improve the biomechanics of the patellofemoral joint, prevention or correction of subluxation is likely to have the most dramatic beneficial effect.

## ANATOMICAL FACTORS IN PATELLOFEMORAL STABILITY

If we are to recognize patellofemoral instability in our patients, then it is important that the anatomical factors favoring patellofemoral stability are well understood. With the leg fully extended and the quadriceps relaxed, the patella is freely mobile with possible medial-lateral passive excursions of a centimeter or more. In this relaxed state with the knee in full extension, the direction of the patellar tendon and the quadriceps tendon form an angle of approximately 15°, the so-called "Q angle." This means that when the quadriceps is tightened there is a

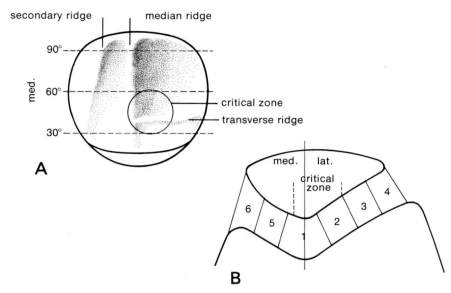

**Figure 3.9.** Anatomical areas of the patellofemoral articular cartilage including the critical zone. Reprinted with permission from Ficat and Hungerford, *Disorders of the Patello-femoral Joint.* Baltimore, Williams & Wilkins, 1977 (7).

valgus vector due to the Q angle (Fig. 3.10). In most individuals this can be easily seen in that quadriceps contraction produces a proximal and slightly lateral movement of the patella as compared to the rest position. As the knee is flexed, the tibia rotates internally, reducing the Q angle and drawing the patella into the trochlear groove. External rotation of the tibia, such as in changing direction of gait, will have the effect of increasing the Q angle and, therefore, increasing the valgus vector. Once the "safe harbor" of the trochlear groove is reached, the patella makes congruent contact with the trochlea as was seen in the contact prints. The PFJR force, therefore, compresses the patella against the congruent trochlea and provides stability. Since the contact area and the PFJR force both increase with increasing flexion, it is perhaps not surprising that most patellofemoral instabilities are manifest in the first 40° of flexion. It is not at all uncommon clinically to see significant subluxation in the 30° flexion film and complete relocation on the 60° film (Fig. 3.11).

Although the valgus vector at the patellofemoral joint probably is the cause of the geographical localization of cartilage

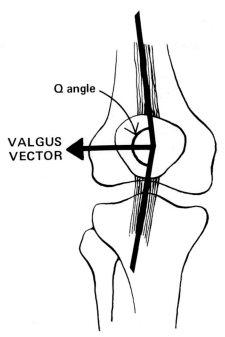

**Figure 3.10.** The Q-angle determines that with quadriceps contraction there will be a laterally directed vector, the "valgus vector."

lesions on the patella, particularly those which progress to full-thickness cartilage loss, it must not be regarded in and of itself as being pathological. The design of the patellofemoral joint with the lateral facet of the trochlea extending more proximally and more anteriorly than the medial facet is shaped to resist lateral patellar subluxation. Also the orientation of the fibers of the vastus medialis, particularly the oblique distal fibers, are aligned to resist lateral subluxation. The actual vector of the combined forces of the quadriceps muscle is a function of the coordinated contraction of its four heads. It is very possible that atrophy of the vastus medialis, particularly following injury or surgery, is responsible for the symptoms in the patellofemoral joint which frequently follow such events. It is also likely that redevelopment of those fibers through quadriceps exercises leads to the reduction in those symptoms as has been seen so often clinically.

In addition the dynamic stabilizers of the patellofemoral joint, there are also static soft tissue stabilizers in the form of the

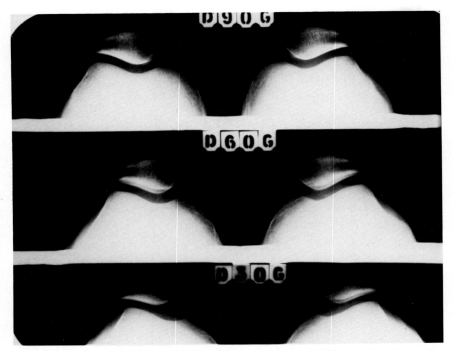

**Figure 3.11.**  A 30°, 60°, and 90° axial view of the patellofemoral joint showing subluxation only at 30°.

patellar tendon, which limits the proximal excursion of the patella when under the influence of quadriceps contraction, and the medial and lateral patellofemoral ligaments, which restrain medial and lateral excursion. Any of these factors may be affected by congenital abnormality, injury, or even surgery.

## ANATOMICAL FACTORS FAVORING PATELLOFEMORAL INSTABILITY

The most common abnormality which has been uncovered in published series of patellofemoral dislocation has been patella alta (6, 11). The most reliable way of measuring patella alta is the ratio of the long axis of the patella to the patellar tendon as seen on the lateral x-ray. Insall and Salvati (12) have determined that 95% of a normal population will have a ratio of patellar tendon to patellar length of less than 1.2. From what we know of the biomechanics and kinematics of the patellofemoral joint, this finding should not be surprising since it means that the patella reaches the safe harbor of the trochlea at a higher degree of knee flexion with a longer patellar tendon. This would mean that the patella would be relatively more at risk of lateral subluxation because the factors which lead to dynamic stability would be operative to a lesser degree in the patient with patella alta at any given degree of knee flexion compared to the normal.

Another anatomical factor favoring patellofemoral instability would be an increase in the Q angle. An increased incidence of patients with a high Q angle has been uncovered not only in series of patellofemoral instability (16), but also in a series of patients with chondromalacia patellae (11). After measuring the Q angle, it is also valuable to check rotation of the hip and the degree of external tibial torsion since femoral anteversion and associated external tibial torsion may be the underlying cause of an increased Q angle. At least some patients with femoral anteversion present with symptoms referable to the patellofemoral joint.

A third factor favoring patellofemoral instability is dysplasia of the patella, the trochlea, or both. This can best be seen on good quality axial views of the patellofemoral views which are recommended for all patients with knee complaints. Finally, the medial and lateral retinaculum should be examined manually by subluxing the patella to the medial or lateral side, respectively, and palpating the retinaculum and the patellofemoral ligaments. Occasionally one will find significant lateral retinacular thickening which may also be a factor in drawing the patella to the lateral side. However, in spite of a diligent search for anatomical factors favoring patellofemoral instability, many patients will be seen in whom no anatomical factor can be uncovered. It must, therefore, be realized that the absence of such discovery does not in the least suggest that the patient in question does not have symptoms on the basis of patellofemoral instability. Many patients will be seen with classic episodes of patellar subluxation and dislocation who are anatomically normal.

## RADIOGRAPHIC SIGNS OF PATELLOFEMORAL INSTABILITY

There are many subtle radiographic signs which are indicative of an instability or an imbalance of forces around the patellofemoral joint. These can only be seen on good quality axial x-rays. Calcification in the medial retinaculum may indicate that this has been mechanically disrupted at the time of a dislocation or significant subluxation (Fig. 3.12). This is literally a give-away sign that can lend objective evidence to a strong clinical suspicion. Axial views in 30° of flexion have already been alluded to as important, since with further flexion, the patella may be perfectly recentered. Lateral retinacular thickening, calcification, or lateral traction osteophytes may indicate an excessive lateral pull by the soft tissue structures. The ELPS has been basically defined by an analysis of the subtle radiographic finding in the absence of evidence of lateral patellar displacement. In addition to the previously mentioned factors, this evidence includes thickening of the subchondral plate and a change in the orientation of the trabecular pattern from perpendicular to the patellar equator to oblique (Fig. 3.13). The presumption is that a combination of dynamic and static forces are tilting the patella to the lateral side. These x-ray signs are

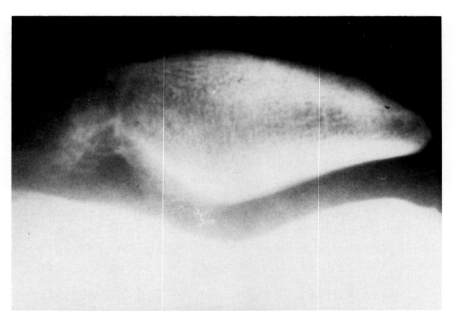

**Figure 3.12.**   Medial retinacular calcification is mute testimony of a prior episode of subluxation or dislocation. Reprinted with permission from Ficat and Hungerford, *Disorders of the Patello-femoral Joint.* Baltimore, Williams & Wilkins, 1977 (7).

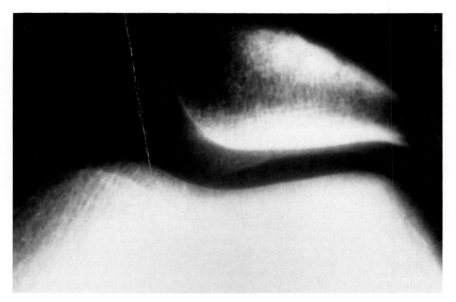

**Figure 3.13.** Subchondral thickening and lateral trabecular orientation suggest excessive lateral pressure.

often associated with indirect or direct evidence of damage to the patellar articular cartilage lateral to the medium ridge and particularly in the area of the critical zone.

## SUMMARY

It appears likely that the changes in unit load which are brought about by lateral subluxation of the patella and also probably by the ELPS are an important mechanism for the breakdown for the patellar articular cartilage which first manifests itself as softening and then deep fibrillation or fasciculation, known as chondromalacia patellae. From autopsy studies and incidental findings at surgery, it is clear that such articular cartilage changes may be evident years and even decades before clinical symptoms. It is also clear from clinical practice that in some individuals this progression can be quite rapid and associated with symptoms earlier than in others. It behooves us as orthopaedic surgeons to look for those factors which favor this diagnosis when encountering a patient with knee complaints. Where possible, those factors should be corrected whether it be through quadriceps rehabilitation, lateral release, tibial tubercle plasty, or proximal realignment, when it can be established that the changes encountered are the cause of the patient's complaints.

## References

1. Aleman O: Chondromalacia post-traumatica patellae. *Acta Chir Scand* 63:194, 1928.
2. Bronitsky J: Chondromalacia patellae. *J Bone Joint Surg* 29:931–945, 1947.
3. Cox FJ: Traumatic osteochondritis of the patella. *Surgery* 17:93–100, 1945.
4. Darracott J, Vernon-Roberts B: The bone changes in "chondromalacia patallae." *Rheumatol Phys Med* 11:175, 1971.
5. Fellander M: Results of chondrectomy in chondromalacia patellae. *Acta Chir Scand* 21:300–318, 1951.
6. Ficat P, Bizou H: Luxations recidivantes de la rotule. *Rev Orthop* 53:721, 1967.
7. Ficat RP, Hungerford DS: *Disorders of the Patello-femoral Joint.* Baltimore, The Williams & Wilkins Co., 1977.
8. Goodfellow JW, Bullough P: The pattern of aging of the articular cartilage of the elbow joint. *J Bone Joint Surg* 49B:175–181, 1967.
9. Hirsch C: A contribution to the pathogenesis of chondromalacia of the patella. Physical, histologic, and chemical study. *Acta Chir Scand* (Suppl.)90:83, 1944.
10. Hungerford DS, Haynes DW: The dynamics of patellar stabilization in knee flexion and rotation. *Trans 28th ORS* 7:254, 1982.
11. Insall J, Falvo KA, Wise DW: Chondromalacia patellae. *J Bone Joint Surg* 58A:1–8, 1976.
12. Insall J, Salvati E: Patella position in the normal knee joint. *Radiology* 101:101–104, 1971.
13. Kallio KE: Chondromalacia patellae. *Ann Chir Gynaecol Fenn* 36:173, 1947.
14. Owre AA: Chondromalacia patallae. *Acta Chir Scand* 77:(Suppl. 41)9, 1936.
15. Robinson AR, Darracott J: Chondromalacia patellae. A survey conducted at the Army Medical Rehabilitation Unit, Chester. *Ann Phys Med* 10:286–290, 1970.
16. Trillat A, Dejour H, Coutette A: Diagnostic et traitement des subluxations recidivantes de la rotule. *Rev Chir Orthop* 50:813–824, 1964.

# CHAPTER FOUR

# Cartilage Lesions and Chondromalacia

**JOHN GOODFELLOW, M.S., F.R.C.S.**

In any discussion of the theoretical basis of chondromalacia patellae, it is first necessary to try to define the meaning of that term and to disentangle it from the numerous inappropriate meanings which it has attracted. Etymologically, it means "softening of the cartilage on the back of the knee cap"; it is a simple descriptive term of morbid anatomy and not the title of a clinical syndrome. There is, in fact, little reason to associate changes in the cartilage on the back of the knee cap with any clinical symptoms whatever, for most of the changes which are referred to exist, to some degree, in most people's knee joints without them being aware of it.

The function of articular cartilage, wherever it occurs, is to resist compressive loading. In order, therefore, to grasp the significance of the patterns of its degeneration we must first understand the pattern of contact which occurs, in life, between the patella and the femur. Figure 4.1 shows how this pattern alters as the knee bends from the fully extended to the fully flexed posture. At first, near full extension, there is only a narrow band of contact, at the inferior pole of the patella. This small area matches the small component of force which is all the patellofemoral joint has to resist when the knee is near extension. At 45° of flexion, the band of contact has moved proximally on the patella and has increased in area, to match the increased compressive force to be expected. At about 90°, or beyond, the band of contact reaches the upper pole of the patella and, by this time, the patella has reached the inferior limit of the trochlear facets on the femur. Somewhere between 100–130° of flexion, the exact angle varying from subject to subject, the patella slides off the trochlear facets and engages the femoral condyles. The *lower diagram* shows how the contact

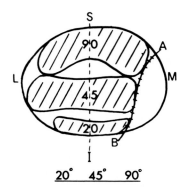

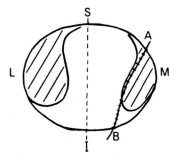

**Figure 4.1.** Diagrammatic representation of contact areas on the patella in varying degrees of flexion. Reprinted with permission from *J Bone Joint Surg* 58B:3, 1976.

areas change. The "odd", or medial longitudinal facet of the patella now articulates with the medial femoral condyle, and the medial facet has become an area of noncontact.

At first sight, it appears that the area available to resist the patellofemoral force is diminished when the patella glides off its trochlear facets and on to the femoral condyles. However, as Figure 4.2 shows, a large area of contact then exists between the posterior surface of the quadriceps tendon and the femur. The patellofemoral force, therefore, can be transmitted, in part, across the tendofemoral joint and, in part, across the patello-femoral joint.

The first conclusion to be drawn from these anatomical facts is that the shapes of the articular surfaces of the patella and those of the femur match one another in a very precise manner. Each contact area, on one surface, matches its fellow on the

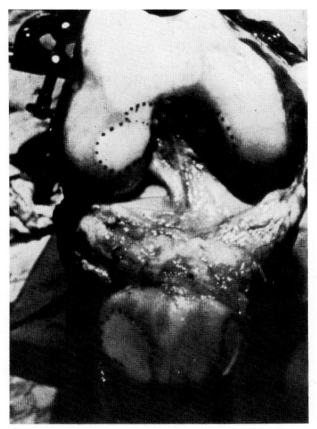

**Figure 4.2.**    Photograph of experiment on the right knee. The extensor mechanism with the patella is turned down so that the femoral and patella contact areas are revealed in 135 degrees of flexion. Reprinted with permission from *J Bone Joint Surg* 58B:3, 1976.

other and this precise fit, at each degree of flexion of the joint, depends upon the precise length and disposition of the soft tissues in which the patella is set. Any alteration in the soft tissue investment of the front of the knee, whether caused by accident, disease, or surgical design must dislocate these contact areas.

A knowledge of the contact areas may also serve to explain the localization of some cartilage lesions. Fibrillation has been known to affect the surface of the odd facet in many young subjects and in most adults for a long time. It seems to be a lesion caused by habitual disuse rather than overuse. The odd facet is only employed when the knee is fully flexed, and that is a position only occasionally adopted by the denizens of an urban society. Surface lesions on the odd facet, though they become almost universal as the population ages, do not progress to the exposure of underlying bone. In their causation and in their course they are similar to other areas of disuse degeneration which have been described in other joints. They are almost certainly symptomless and their presence, in the knee of a patient complaining of pain, must not be misinterpreted as the cause of that pain.

By contrast, within the areas of habitual contact, cartilage degeneration is likely to progress. As cartilage fails under mechanical load, the signs and symptoms of osteoarthritis may eventually develop. However, symptoms are seldom present before degeneration has progressed to the frank exposure of underlying bone, which is why patellofemoral arthritis is a disorder of the middle-aged and the elderly and is seldom an explanation for pain in the young knee.

If neither of these patterns of degeneration occasions pain in youth, is there, perhaps, another disorder, peculiar to the patellofemoral articulation, which can cause aching pain in the young knee? A cartilage lesion quite unlike the foregoing degenerations has been reported in young patients suffering from knee pain. It is not a surface degeneration but a change which initially involves only the deeper layers of the cartilage. Figure 4.3 shows, diagrammatically, the lesion which we have called "fasciculation", to distinguish it from the surface degeneration called fibrillation.

This lesion has been observed, predominately astride the median ridge of the patella, and astride the ridge which separates the medial from the odd facet, in many young subjects complaining of anterior knee pain. This by no means proves that the lesion is the cause of the pain, for we do not know how often it occurs in joints which are asymptomatic. There is, however, some circumstantial evidence to suggest that, unlike the two cartilage lesions just discussed, it could be a source of pain.

Firstly, the disorganization of the midzone of the cartilage might give rise to pain, experienced through nerve endings in the subchondral bone, when pressure is applied. We know that

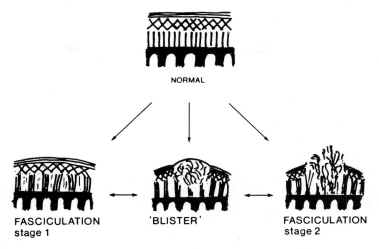

**Figure 4.3.** Stages in the lesion of basal degeneration. Reprinted with permission from *J Bone Joint Surg* 58B:3, 1976.

the lattice of collagen in this zone alters its orientation under load and that it probably acts as an energy absorber.

Secondly, such a lesion could exist in a joint for a long period of time without producing any of the signs of arthritis. Since, in this lesion, the articular surface is the last to fail, effusion into the joint need not be expected. Such a disorder could cause pain in certain postures of the knee, and not in others, and it could continue for many years and yet occasion no secondary changes whatever.

Lastly, such a lesion might be reversible, at least until the point of rupture of the lamina splendens was reached.

The classical features of the clinical syndrome of anterior knee pain, its long duration, the absence of physical signs, and its strong tendency to recover spontaneously may all be thus explained.

Occasionally, the lesion progresses to rupture of the tangential surface layer (Fig. 4.4) and then an effusion appears in the joint, often containing innumerable free particles of shed cartilage. Such cases are rare, but those that I have seen have not complained of pain. The ruptured lesion would not be capable of transmitting high loads to the bone beneath and so, again, the mechanics of the lesion match the physical signs.

In other parts of this symposium, the case will be argued for

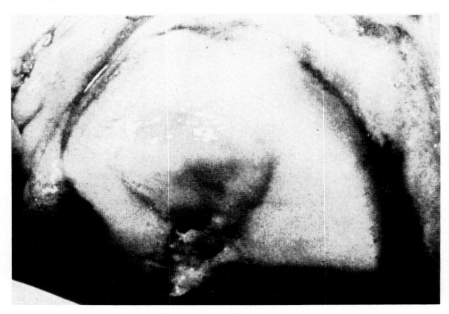

**Figure 4.4.** Photograph at operation of a lesion astride the ridge between the odd and medial facets. It is confluent with a second area astride the median ridge. The patient had a large effusion in the knee and the synovial fluid contained innumerable fragments of shed cartilage. Histological examination revealed the lesion to consist of fibrous tissue which had repaired, inadequately, the large defect from which the cartilage had been shed. Reprinted with permission from *J Bone Joint Surg* 58B:3, 1976.

this or that, intra-articular or extra-articular cause for the enigmatic symptom of chronic anterior knee pain in young people. It is my purpose firstly to draw attention to my belief that most cartilage lesions, particularly those which are visible, either at arthrotomy or through the arthroscope, are irrelevant. Surface degenerative changes are probably symptomless, unless or until they expose bone. But a certain cartilage lesion, which afflicts the midzone of the cartilage and which we call fasciculation, may cause pain in some young knees. Except in those rare cases in which it bursts through to the surface, it must be presumed to be capable of spontaneous recovery. Its presence, therefore, would certainly not justify its destruction either by "shaving" or by excision.

# CHAPTER FIVE

# Can Articular Cartilage Heal?

RUDOLF LEMPERG, M.D., PH.D.

The question in the title appears at first glance to be quite easy to answer: 1) intracartilaginous defects will not heal and 2) osteocartilaginous defects will (may) heal. These statements are based on the prevailing conclusions made in the relevant international literature (1–4, 6, 7, 9, 10, 13, 15, 20, 22, 31, 32, 34–36, 42, 45) on these subjects and also on my own observations (15, 25, 27).

However, at second glance, the correctness of these statements appears to be dubious with regard to the real meaning of the word "heal" as far as hyaline articular cartilage is concerned. The implication of heal must first be strictly clarified not only because of semantics, but also in order to assort the various observations published as to their proximity to healing of the articular cartilage.

In *The Random House Dictionary of the English Language* (38), the following is found under heal (irrelevant alternatives are omitted):

1. to make whole or sound, restore to health, free from ailment;

2. to free from evil;

3. to effect a cure;

4. (of a wound, broken bone, etc.) to become whole or sound.

Applying heal to hyaline articular cartilage on a joint surface cannot be interpreted strictly as anything less than "restoring the articular surface with hyaline cartilage", and if a defect on the articular surface is encountered as well, "restoring the surface to normal level." One other alternative could possibly be accepted. Also other tissue which is "sound" or which has "effected a cure" could be said to have healed an articular cartilage defect. In this case, the permanency of the effected cure has to be proved since normal hyaline cartilage certainly does last under normal conditions for a whole lifetime.

Reading certain literature about healing of articular cartilage defects gives one the suspicion that "free from evil" (alternative 2 in the *Random House Dictionary*) was the definition used for assessment of the type of cartilage healing. The interested reader should consult the *Synonym Finder* (39) for further clarification of evil—however, it will certainly not facilitate the understanding of the nature of the cartilage healing process.

In order to avoid further confusion, strict adherence to the subjects of healing of 1) intracartilaginous defects and 2) osteochondral defects on articular surfaces of diarthrodial mammalian joints is necessary. Concerning osteochondral defects, the repair of the joint surface with cartilaginous tissue will be addressed. Special attention will be paid to the interrelationship between the type of articular surface tissue and restoration of a continuous subchondral bone plate and further to the influence of motion and immobilization on the differentiation process of the tissue constituting the joint surface.

## ANATOMICAL REMARKS

In adult mammals, the hyaline articular cartilage rests on a continuous subchondral bone plate with characteristics of a cortical shell (25, 30) which, however, in limited areas, consists only of a thin lamellar bone layer (25). On this subchondral bone plate, the calcified cartilage layer rests, which, in turn, is separated by the tidemark (12) from the noncalcified articular cartilage. The tidemark is kept at an almost constant distance from the articular surface throughout life, with a very slow advancement of mineralization toward the joint (25) (Fig. 5.1). There appears to be a delicate physiological system in the articular cartilage probably governed by gradients of solutes (33) and matrix constituents (28, 33) which maintain this constant calcification-front and also prevent the vessels from subchondral bone invading the calcified cartilage (36, 44). The presence of an intact subchondral bone plate covered by normal articular cartilage is probably also of importance for the energy absorbing property of the joint ends of the long bones (37).

## INTRACARTILAGINOUS DEFECTS IN ARTICULAR CARTILAGE

It appears that there is general agreement that intracartilaginous defects will remain largely unaltered over a long

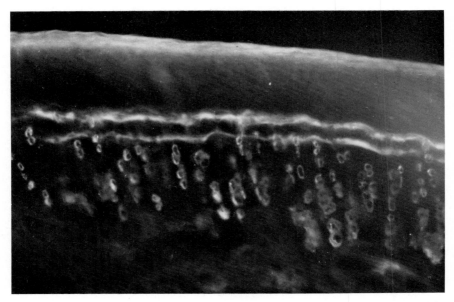

**Figure 5.1.** Fluorescence photomicrograph from the femoral head of an adult rabbit. The animal was labeled twice with tetracycline with an interval of 7 months. The animal was 9 months old at the first labeling; the second labeling was given 2 days before death. The fluorescent line closer to the articular surface can be attributed to second labeling while the labeling closer to the subchondral bone is from the first labeling. This picture indicates slow progression of the calcification front towards the joint. Reprinted with permission from Lemperg R, *Virchows Arch Abt A Path Anat* 352:14–25, 1971 (25).

period of time (Fig. 5.2) and certainly not be filled out by tissue emanating from the articular cartilage itself. This is certainly true for adult individuals but seems also to be the rule in young mammals (9). There are some reports (4, 10) which describe the occurrence of limited new cartilage formation in defects on the joint surface of growing animals. However, this is to be seen as an exception to the rule. In adult mammals, it has never been proved that proliferation of chondrocytes in the articular cartilage itself increases the bulk of the cartilage tissue and, thus, contributes to filling of a defect in the cartilage. What has been shown is that 3H-thymidine is incorporated in chondrocytes (9, 10, 24, 29, 30) indicating mitotic cell division after damage to the cartilage. A 3H-thymidine-labeled mitosis in a chondrocyte was published as early as 1967 by Lemperg (24). What may or may not occur in intracartilaginous defects is

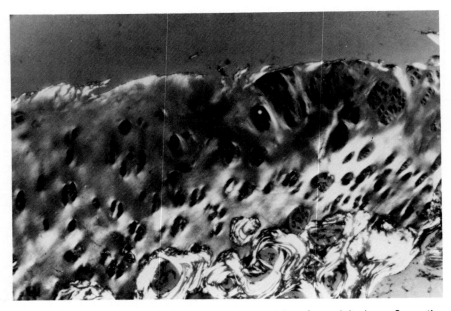

**Figure 5.2.**  Intracartilaginous defect in the knee joint of an adult sheep 6 months after removal of the tangential layer on a femoral condyle in an area of 0.5 × 0.75 cm. The joint was not immobilized after the operation and the sheep was kept outdoors on a farm during the entire observation period. Photomicrograph of hematoxylin-eosin-stained decalcified section in polarized light. To the *left*, the superficial layer of the cartilage is devoid of chondrocytes and the surface shows superficial fibrillation. The fibrillated area shows also polarization effect as a sign that collagen is partly exposed due to loss of proteoglycans. To the *right*, several multinuclear chondrones containing a large amount of nuclei are seen—in this area, stronger stainability of intercellular substance is visible as sign of proteoglycan production. The joint surface over this area shows only minimal polarization effect and appears smoother. The cellular reaction of the chondrocytes, thus, can be two-fold; they might die or multiply within one chondrone.

nevertheless of interest since proper understanding of this process will give some guidance also for our view on the initiation and progress of osteoarthritis—as far as osteoarthritis is a disease of the joint surface.

In Figure 5.2, four typical phenomena associated with intracartilaginous defects can be seen within a limited area. These are:

1. depletion of the defect margin of chondrocytes;
2. multinuclear chondrones in the defect margin;
3. fibrillation of the surface with prominent collagen fibers (in area with chondrocyte depletion);

4. smooth surface, without fibrillation and with restored matrix stainability (in area with multinuclear chondrones).

Further, it should be noted that there is no pannus tissue visible on the articular surface. The defect shown is 6 months after removal of the tangential layer of the cartilage within a 0.5 × 0.75 cm area with a scalpel, centrally on the femoral condyle of an adult sheep knee joint. This animal was never immobilized after the operation.

The type of experimental model not only influences the morphological appearance of an individual intracartilaginous defect but also the metabolic response of the cartilage itself and the underlying subchondral bone.

## Cartilage Observation

Scarification (7, 29, 34, 45) will create a rather deep defect in the cartilage with smooth cut surfaces but it will not remove any major portion of the tangential layer. This layer is believed to have not only a protective biological (27, 36) but also a mechanical function (5, 37) for the deeper parts of the cartilage. Removal of the tangential layer in a larger surface area (3, 4, 10, 20, 26, 27, 35, 36) will expose major parts of the bulk of the cartilage to the influence of synovial fluid (19) and, thus, the opportunity to introduce major metabolic alterations in the chondrocytes. It also may alter the mechanical property of the remaining cartilage and also the stress pattern of the underlying bone (5, 37). This might explain some differences between scarification and surface area defects both with regard to observations on the remaining cartilage and in the reaction of the subchondral bone (26, 27) to the cartilage defects.

The rim of cartilage without living chondrocytes along the border of the defect (Fig. 5.3) is common to all types of defects and is well documented in most publications. However, fibrillation of the articular surface (Fig. 5.4) with demascation of collagen fibers, loss of proteoglycans, and resembling the picture in human osteoarthritis, as a rule, will not become visible in scarification models.

Pannus tissue on the joint surface of the defect will preferably occur as a consequence of immobilization (45). Moreover, immobilization might introduce irreversible cartilage damage

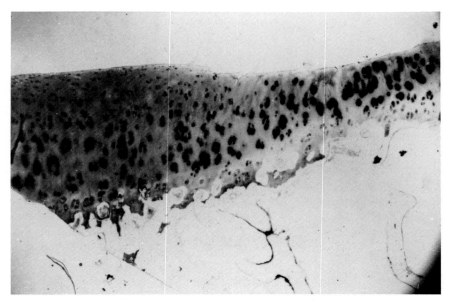

**Figure 5.3.** Autoradiograph after 35S-sulphate labeling in vitro of superficial articular cartilage defect. Observe the lack of labeled chondrocytes along the border of the defect and also in deeper layers of the cartilage beneath the defect area. Autoradiograph stained with toluidine blue.

(11, 41, 43, 45). On the other hand motion, passive (42) or active (9), will favorably influence the articular cartilage.

Whether an intracartilaginous defect is situated on a weight-bearing surface or on a nonweight-bearing seems not to affect its long-term appearance (9). However, it is affected by a peripheral localization close to perichondrium or synovial tissue from where pannus tissue may arise and over it (10).

Since matrix flow into defect margins is well known to occur and since this phenomenon might easily be misinterpreted as healing, serial section of entire defect areas appears to be one important methodological consideration when studying superficial cartilage defects. Sixty years ago, serial sectioning was strongly advocated by Haebler (13) in every case where mesenchymal tissue was observed in intracartilaginous defects because violation of the subchondral bone would be found in each instance. This recommendation is still valid today.

Among approaches to influence beneficially on the healing of cartilage defects, it is worth mentioning hyaluronic acid

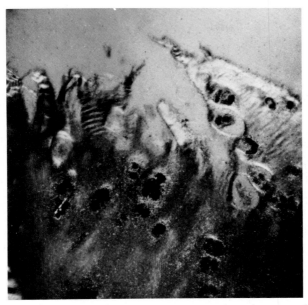

**Figure 5.4.** Detail from a superficial articular cartilage defect in an adult sheep after 6 months of observation (same as Fig. 5.2). Autoradiograph after 35S-sulphate labeling seen in polarized light. Demascation of collagen within the fibrillated surface is clearly visible. Labeled chondrocytes are found in close vicinity to the fibrillation clefts. The photographic emulsion is seen as white grains in polarized light. Reprinted with permission from Lemperg et al., *Virchows Arch Abt A Path Anat* 354:1–17, 1971 (27).

application into joints since it is a rather recent whim. However, it has been shown, not surprisingly, that it has no effect whatsoever on healing (45).

## Subchondral Bone Reaction

The occurrence of sclerosis in the subchondral area as part of the osteoarthritic picture generally is accepted. However, the early response of the subchondral bone to limited intracartilaginous defects is less well documented. Histological studies will not easily disclose small subchondral bone alterations but tetracycline labeling in vivo will give a dynamic picture of the calcified subchondral structure. Figure 5.5 shows an intracartilaginous defect in an adult rabbit femoral head 2 weeks after surgery with intense fluorescence (active calcification) in the tidemark area under the defect. The

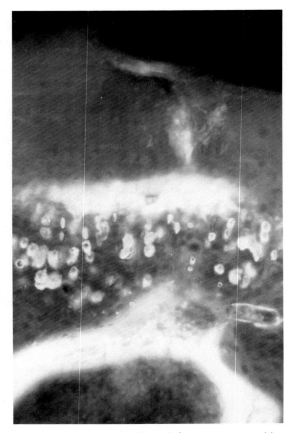

**Figure 5.5.**  A superficial articular cartilage defect was created in an adult rabbit and the animal was labeled with tetracycline 12 days after the operation; 2 days later the animal was sacrificed (same animal as Fig. 5.6). The photomicrograph shows an undecalcified section in ultraviolet light. Heavy fluorescence, indicating active calcification is seen in the tidemark directly beneath the defect area. The subchondral bone lamella shows also heavy fluorescence. Observe that articular cartilage covers the fluorescent area. Reprinted with permission from Lemperg R, *Virchows Arch Abt A Path Anat* 354:14–25, 1971 (26).

microradiogram (Fig. 5.6) of the identical area shows that obviously mineral was lost. The vigorous calcification, thus, is interpretable as a response to previous local loss of mineral. After 6 months, an intracartilaginous defect in the femoral condyle of an adult sheep shows a small subchondral osteophyte, still with active mineralization in the tidemark but strictly localized to the defect area (Fig. 5.7).

These observations were previously reported in detail (26, 27)

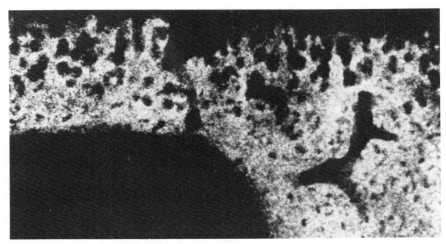

**Figure 5.6.** Microradiograph from identical section and area shown in Figure 5.5. In the corresponding area shown in Figure 5.5, intense fluorescence loss of mineral is clearly seen in this picture. Figures 5.5 and 5.6 together indicate that mineral in the calcified cartilage is lost early as a response to an intracartilaginous defect. This loss is immediately inducing a new calcification. This calcification might, however, proceed further towards the joint surface than the initial tidemark was situated. Reprinted with permission from Lemperg R, *Virchows Arch Abt A Path Anat* 354:14–25, 1971 (26).

and can be interpreted so that the earliest reactions of the mineralized subchondral structure are loss of mineral around subchondral vessels, in the tidemark, and adjacent calcified cartilage layer and that reactive calcification and eventually bone formation occurs thereafter. This active calcification might result in an advancement of the calcification front toward the joint surface and subsequently in local osteophyte formation. These alterations are strictly localized to the area of intracartilaginous defect and may be interpreted safely as a consequence of the primary cartilage defect. Whether such subchondral osteophytes finally result in a progressive lesion of type "experimental osteoarthritis", perhaps due to alterations of mechanical properties of the overlying cartilage, is an open question.

## OSTEOCHONDRAL LESIONS

The knowledge of healing of osteochondral defects by cartilage-resembling tissue is a century old and the literature of

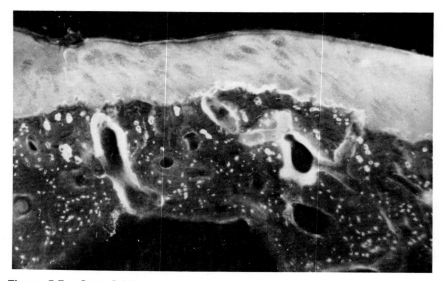

**Figure 5.7.** Superficial articular cartilage defect in adult sheep after 6 months. (This animal was treated similar to the one shown in Fig. 5.2). The animal received tetracycline 2 days prior to death. Microphotograph of undecalcified section in ultraviolet light. In the remaining articular cartilage, numerous multinuclear chondrones are visible. Beneath this area, a subchondral osteophyte has developed which still is showing in parts intense fluorescence, indicating active calcification. In the subchondral bone plate, numerous bone surfaces show fluorescence, indicating remodeling of the bone plate. Reprinted with permission from Lemperg et al., *Virchows Arch Abt A Path Anat* 354:1–17, 1971 (27).

that time is cited frequently (3, 6, 7, 9, 10, 31). One issue which had been vigorously discussed during decades—the source of the cell population filling the defect—was essentially solved in 1966 by the work of DePalma et al. (9) using 3H-thymidine autoradiography. It was shown convincingly that the defect was filled by cells emanating from the subchondral bone which—by metaplasia—could with time resemble, morphologically, cartilage tissue. The articular cartilage adjacent to the defect margins showed few labeled chondrocytes which, however, did not in any way contribute to the cell population filling the defect. This observation was true for both growing and adult dogs and it is also consistent with observations by others (10, 18, 32) using 3H-thymidine technique.

The other item which has excited researchers is whether hyaline cartilage eventually will fill such a defect or if it is some type of fibrocartilage.

Before microchemical techniques were available, the characterization of hyaline cartilage rested upon purely morphological methods which have clearly limited accuracy for this purpose. The proof of the presence of hyaline cartilage must nowadays be corroborated by combining morphological with chemical techniques. However, it has been shown that chemical alterations may precede morphologically visible changes (16) in articular cartilage which makes the combination of both techniques more important than ever. Using this approach, Akeson et al. (1) in 1968 showed that regenerates on the surface of the femoral head after removal of entire articular cartilage down to the subchondral bone in dogs never reached total hexosamine concentrations similar to those of normal articular cartilage (total hexosamines 3.5% per dry weight and 4.6%, respectively). The collagen content in contrast was higher in the regenerates, which is characteristic of fibrocartilage. The qualitative analyses of proteoglycan constituents showed certain similarity to hyaline cartilage. These findings are consistent with our own microchemical data obtained from rabbit hip joints (15). This chemical study (15) was carried out on freeze-dried sections after microdissection of the material and morphological characterization of each sample. Therefore, for each chemically studied sample the individual morphological structure was known—a method never used before on such material—and unfortunately not often used since then. Table 5.1 shows the course of differentiation, with increasing time, in osteochondral defects as seen in the light microscope and expressed as a proportion of keratan sulphate to chondroitin sulphate. In Figure 5.8, the keratan sulphate and chondroitin sulphate contents per dry weight are expressed as percentage of the articular cartilage in the same animal. In Figure 5.9, an autoradiographical picture of a defect area is shown after observation of 12 weeks. Table 5.1 shows that the relative content of chondroitin sulphate increases with increasing proportion of cartilaginous tissue in the defect. (For definitions of the type of tissue observed, the original paper should be read.) Chemically the greatest similarity with articular cartilage is achieved after 8–12 weeks, at which time also a morphological and metabolic similarity exists. However, in accordance with the finding of Akeson et al., the total hexosamine content does not reach the same level in the regenerate as it

**Table 5.1.**
**Osteochondral Defect on the Femoral Head of 1-year-old Rabbits**

| Animal No. | Obs. Times Weeks | Hexosamines | | Type of tissue | |
|---|---|---|---|---|---|
| | | 1 % CPC | 0.6 M MgCl$_2$ | Connective Tissue | Cartilaginous |
| 382 | 1 | 55.3 | 16.9 | +++ | |
| 383 | 1 | 56.1 | 20.6 | +++ | |
| 384 | 1 | 62.3 | 15.1 | +++ | |
| 372 | 2 | 58.2 | 23.9 | ++ | + |
| 374 | 2 | 50.7 | 29.2 | +++ | |
| 385 | 2 | 41.2 | 45.8 | +(+) | +(+) |
| 367 | 4 | 52.7 | 33.5 | ++ | + |
| 368 | 4 | 45.9 | 32.9 | + | ++ |
| 369 | 4 | 51.0 | 34.1 | ++ | + |
| 418 | 4 | 50.1 | 34.8 | + | ++ |
| 361 | 8 | 33.2 | 55.5 | | +++ |
| 362 | 8 | 42.5 | 40.3 | + | ++ |
| 363 | 8 | 33.8 | 56.8 | | +++ |
| 356 | 12 | lost | — | + | ++ |
| 357 | 12 | 37.1 | 44.5 | | +++ |
| 358 | 12 | 40.5 | 43.2 | | +++ |
| 350 | 20 | 40.4 | 47.1 | | +++ |
| 352 | 20 | 54.1 | 27.8 | ++(+) | (+) |
| 353 | 20 | 49.7 | 32.1 | ++ | + |
| 344 | 40 | 36.8 | 51.8 | | +++ |
| 349 | 40 | 41.5 | 35.2 | (+) | ++(+) |
| 340 | 40 | 48.1 | 32.1 | ++ | + |
| 338 | 52 | 32.1 | 57.8 | | +++ |
| 342 | 52 | 34.4 | 26.6 | ++(+) | (+) |

Percentage distribution of hexosamines in the 1% CPC (keratan sulphate + glycoproteins) and 0.6 M MgCl$_2$ (chondroitin sulphate) fractions from cellulose columns and the morphological appearance on azure A-stained freeze-dried sections from the defect area.

The amount of hexosamines in the two fractions is expressed as percentage of total hexosamines eluted from the columns during the procedure (15) and does not add up to 100%. Each + indicates approximately one-third of the defect area composed of that type of tissue. Reprinted with permission from Hjertquist and Lemberg (15), see Figure 5.8 also.

does in articular cartilage of the same animal. Thus, a morphological similarity contrasts to a much lesser chemical resemblance.

The third item of great importance is the observation that secondary degeneration will occur frequently in regenerates after more than 6 months (1, 9, 15, 35). The occurrence of this phenomenon has not been described too frequently simply because few researchers observe their animals long enough. However, this secondary degeneration is a long-term threat to the

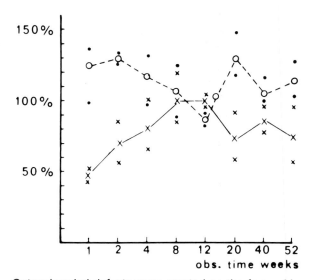

xXx Mg Cl₂ fraction

•o• 1% CPC fraction

**Figure 5.8.** Osteochondral defects were created on the femoral head of 1-year-old rabbits. The animals were not immobilized after surgery. The femoral heads were frozen at −76° Celsius and subsequently 40 thick frozen sections were prepared and freeze-dried. The defect area and the articular cartilage were separately dissected out and subsequently fractionated on cellulose columns using the CPC technique (15). The 1% CPC fraction represents keratan sulphate plus glycoprotein and the MgCl₂ fraction chondroitin sulphate.

The figure shows the change of these glycosaminoglycans in the defect tissue with time. The values in the defect tissue are calculated as a percentage of those in the articular cartilage in the same animal. The mean values from all animals in a group are shown and the highest and lowest value. Note that the greatest similarity to the articular cartilage is reached at 12 weeks when also a small scatter of values is found. Reprinted with permission from Hjertquist and Lemperg, *Calc Tiss Res* 8:54–72, 1971 (15).

regenerate, especially if the level of the subchondral bone is advanced towards the joint surface with progressive thinning of the cartilage tissue (Fig. 5.10) as a consequence.

Some factors are known to influence the differentiation process of the regenerate tissue. Immobilization will have a negative effect upon differentiation toward cartilage. Additionally, it might jeopardize the surface tissue by stimulating the invasion of subchondral vessels into the calcified cartilage (11, 32, 41, 45).

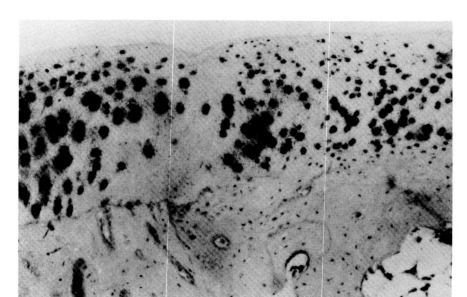

**Figure 5.9.** Osteochondral defect on the femoral head of a 1-year-old rabbit after 12 weeks. Autoradiograph after 35S-sulphate labeling. The normal articular cartilage to the *left*, the defect area to the *right*. There is a border layer of tissue between the two areas without labeled chondrocytes. The chondrocytes in the defect area show similar sulphate uptake as the articular cartilage. Reprinted with permission from Hjertquist and Lemperg, *Calc Tiss Res* 8:54–72, 1971 (15).

Most authors agree that maintained joint function appears to be beneficial. Early passive motion was claimed to be beneficial for healing of osteochondral defects (42). However, in this paper, the estimation of the presence of hyaline cartilage was based solely on light microscopy. The microphotographs said to represent hyaline cartilage are not too representative and easily could be designated as immature cartilage. The beneficial effect of the passive motion was substantiated, unfortunately, by comparison with a control group which obviously showed an excessive low spontaneous occurrence of cartilaginous tissue in the defect. Whatever early passive motion might mean for tissue differentiation to hyaline cartilage in osteochondral defects—this particular paper has certainly not ascertained it.

The size of the defect is apparently of importance. Large defects which do not protect the regenerates and provide suitable mechanical prerequisites will produce poorer conditions for

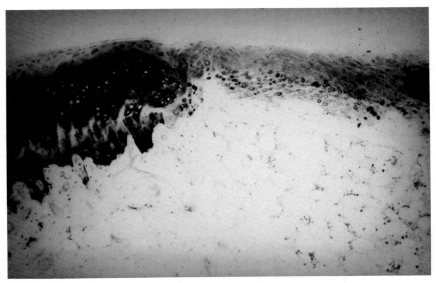

**Figure 5.10.** Osteochondral defect on femoral head of adult rabbit after 52 weeks. To the *right*, the defect area is covered by tissue with morphological appearance of hyaline cartilage. There is a distinct layer of calcified cartilage. The surface layer shows poor stainability, fewer chondrocytes, and, in places, some fibrillation. The cartilage is much thinner than the articular cartilage to the *right*. The picture strongly suggests degenerative changes in the regenerate.

differentiation as do very narrow ones—which lack mechanical stimuli. Defects with a size of approximately 3 × 3 mm seem to be optimal for differentiation studies. Most authors, including myself, describe frequently "incomplete filling" of defects—in these instances, the tissue will be of the fibrous type besides cartilaginous tissue of varying differentiation grades.

Since mechanical factors certainly influence the differentiation process, one interesting observation was made by myself (15)—cartilaginous tissue of mature appearance would not occur unless the subchondral bone plate in the base of the defect was restored and the marrow cavities were sealed by bony tissue. Probably the restored subchondral bone plate supports the regenerate tissue and acts as pressure distributor giving the correct differentiation stimulus. In the same paper (15), another observation was reported which should perhaps have some bearing on the healing process. Differentiation toward cartilaginous tissue did not progress ad infinitum, but it seemed that tissue which had not matured by 3 months would not differentiate further but stay at that level. In contrast, DePalma et al. reported maturation of cartilaginous tissue up to more than 1 year of follow-up.

Observations on autologous costal cartilage transplanted to osteochondral defects on the femoral head and observed up to 1½ years (16) would support the views of the importance of sealing of the medullary cavities and also the limited time span during which differentiation actually will occur. Moreover, also in this study no real chemical similarity between defect tissue and articular cartilage was found in spite of excessive observation times and the presence undoubtedly of hyaline cartilage (16, 17).

## COMMENTS

There are some peculiarities in articular cartilage which should be considered when talking about the possibility of healing of this tissue. Three of these peculiarities I have chosen to mention briefly.

First: the mechanical properties of the articular cartilage versus subchondral bone constitute a fine balanced system where the intrinsic mechanical property of the cartilage is of great importance (40). It has been shown that articular cartilage stiffness is correlated to total proteoglycan content rather than to collagen content (21). Further, proteoglycan content was found to be correlated to cartilage elasticity (14, 23). Since it has been demonstrated that proteoglycans (hexosamines), as a rule, will not reach normal values in regenerates, altered mechanical properties are to be expected. Anyone who has seen and grossly felt the consistency of cartilaginous regenerates after an osteo-cartilaginous defect on a joint surface would agree with me that the mechanical property of these regenerates must be grossly different from the original cartilage. One study, in fact, has demonstrated that compression properties of articular cartilage and regenerates are different (8). Studies where chemical and mechanical properties are determined properly on morphologically characterized tissue are still awaited. Preferably also the effect of joint motion on regenerates could be studied using such combinations of methods.

Second: the delicate distribution of water, proteoglycans, collagen, and glycoproteins throughout the cartilage with gradients from the joint surface toward the subchondral bone are essential for transport of solutes to and from the chondrocytes. Disturbance of these gradients will not only affect the chondrocyte metabolism and eventually cause degeneration of the tissue but also activate the cells in the subchondral vessels prompting bone resorption or formation. It seems to me that no scar tissue ever could regain this fine organization level of the original cartilage. No microchemical studies have been made yet to study regenerates with these aspects in mind.

Third: in contrast to costal cartilage, which has been shown to have the ability of intrinsic proliferation of chondrocytes with new production of substantial amounts of cartilage tissue (24), the articular cartilage lacks this capability. Since both articular cartilage and costal cartilage are hyaline cartilage, the fact of being this type of tissue alone cannot be the reason for the lack of the former to intrinsic proliferation. The frequently observed multinuclear chondrones in damaged articular cartilage are certainly a product of mitotic chondrocyte division, but they do not contribute in any way to increase the bulk of the cartilage tissue. What could be the reason for this difference? One possible explanation is that nature does not want any remodeling of articular cartilage on a tissue level since it could disturb both the mechanical properties of the cartilage and the gradient system which provide the prerequisite for the nutrient flow. In this concept would also fit the fact that cartilage does have an extensive remodeling of matrix—constituents which will not tend to alter the tissue structure but will renew the carriers of the physico-chemical properties.

## CONCLUSION

Articular cartilage defects in adult individuals will not heal by hyaline cartilage having mechanical and chemical properties equal to normal articular cartilage. This is true for osteochondral defects but also for superficial, intracartilaginous defects. Osteochondral defects will be filled by scar tissue which by metaplasia, beneficially influenced by joint motion, may develop toward cartilaginous tissue of varying maturation degree. However, secondary degeneration and possibly progressive subchondral bone changes will be a continuous threat to these regenerates.

**References**

1. Akeson WH, Miyashita C, Taylor TKF, et al: Experimental arthroplasty of the canine hip. *J Surg Res* 8:26–40, 1968.
2. Bennet GA, Bauer W: Further studies concerning the repair of articular cartilage in dog joints. *J Bone Joint Surg* 17:141–150, 1935.
3. Bucher U: Befunde nach experimentellen gelenkknorpeldefekten beim meerschweinchen. *Schweiz Z Path* 18:185–197, 1955.
4. Calandruccio RA, Gilmer WS: Proliferation, regeneration, and repair of articular cartilage of immature animals. *J Bone Joint Surg* 44-A:431–455, 1962.
5. Camosso ME: Analisi del comportamento meccanico delle cartilagini articolari sottoposte a carico. *Boll Soc Ital Biol Sper* 34:331–333, 1958.
6. Campbell CJ: The healing of cartilage defects. *Clin Orthop* 64:45–63, 1969.
7. Carlsson H: Reactions of rabbit patellary cartilage following operative defects. *Acta Orthop Scand* Suppl. 28, 1957.
8. Coletti JM, Akeson WH, Woo SL-Y: A comparison of the physical behavior of normal articular cartilage and the arthroplasty surface. *J Bone Joint Surg* 54-A:147–160, 1972.
9. DePalma AF, McKeever CD, Subin DK: Process of repair of articular cartilage demonstrated by histology and autoradiography with tritiated thymidine. *Clin Orthop* 48:229–242, 1966.
10. Dustmann HO, Puhl W: Altersabhängige heilungsmöglichkeiten von knorpelwunden. Tierexperimentelle untersuchungen. *Z Orthop* 114:749–764, 1976.
11. Evans EB, Eggers GWN, Butler JK, et al: Experimental immobilization and remobilization of rat knee joints. *J Bone Joint Surg* 42-A:737–758, 1960.
12. Fawns HT, Landells JW: Histochemical studies of rheumatic conditions. I. Observations on the fine structures of the matrix of normal bone and cartilage. *Ann Rheum Dis* 12:105–113, 1953.
13. Haebler C: Experimentelle untersuchungen über die regeneration des gelenkknorpels. *Bruns Beitr Klin Chir* 134:602–640, 1925.
14. Hirsch C: A contribution to the pathogenesis of chondromalacia of the patella. *Acta Chir Scand* Suppl. 90, 1944.
15. Hjertquist SO, Lemperg R: Histological, autoradiographic and microchemical studies of spontaneously healing osteochondral articular defects in adult rabbits. *Calc Tiss Res* 8:54–72, 1971.
16. Hjertquist SO, Lemperg R: Long-term observation on the articular cartilage and autologous costal cartilage transplanted to osteochondral defects on the femoral head. *Calc Tiss Res* 9:226–237, 1972.
17. Hjertquist SO, Lemperg R: Microchemical studies on glycosaminoglycans and calcium in autologous costal cartilage transplanted to an osteochondral defect on the femoral head of adult rabbits. *Calc Tiss Res* 5:153–169, 1970.
18. Hjertquist SO, Lemperg R: Transplantation of autologous costal cartilage to an osteochondral defect on the femoral head. Histological and autoradiographical studies in adult rabbits after administration of 35S-sulphate and 3H-thymidine. *Virchows Arch Abt A Path Anat* 346:345–360, 1969.
19. Howell DS, Sapolsky AI, Pita JC, et al: The pathogenesis of osteoarthritis. *Semin Arthritis Rheum* 5:365–383, 1976.
20. Imerlishvili, JA: Experimental study of joint cartilage regeneration. (In Russian) *Arkh Anat (Moskva)* 34:58–71, 1957.
21. Kempson GE, Muir H, Swanson SAV, et al: Correlations between stiffness and the chemical constituents of cartilage on the human femoral head. *Biochim Biophys Acta* 215:70–77, 1970.
22. Key JA: Experimental arthritis: The changes in joints produced by creating defects in the articular cartilage. *J Bone Joint Surg* 13:725–739, 1931.
23. Kopta JA, Blosser JA: Elasticity of articular cartilage. Effects of intra-articular steroid administration and medial meniscectomy. *Clin Orthop* 64:21–32, 1969.
24. Lemperg R: Studies of autologous diced costal cartilage transplant. IV. With special regard to 3H-thymidine incorporation in vitro after intramuscular and further transplantation to the hip joint. *Acta Soc Med Upsal* 72:199–222, 1967.

25. Lemperg R: The subchondral bone plate of the femoral head in adult rabbits. I. Spontaneous remodelling studied by microradiography and tetracycline labelling. *Virchows Arch Abt A Path Anat* 352:1–13, 1971.
26. Lemperg R: The subchondral bone plate of the femoral head in adult rabbits. II. Changes induced by intracartilaginous defects studied by microradiography and tetracycline labelling. *Virchows Arch Abt A Path Anat* 352:14–25, 1971.
27. Lemperg R, Boquist L, Rosenquist J: Intracartilaginous defects in adult sheep. Histological, autoradiographical (35S-sulphate), ultrastructural, microradiographical and fluorochromic studies. *Virchows Arch Abt A Path Anat* 354:1–16, 1971.
28. Lemperg R, Larsson SE, Hjertquist SO: The glycosaminoglycans of bovine articular cartilage. I. Concentration and distribution in different layers in relation to age. *Calc Tiss Res* 15:237–251, 1974.
29. Mankin HJ: Localization of tritiated thymidine in articular cartilage of rabbits. II. Repair in immature cartilage. *J Bone Joint Surg* 44-A:688–698, 1966.
30. Mankin HJ: Localization of tritiated thymidine in articular cartilage of rabbits. III. Mature articular cartilage. *J Bone Joint Surg* 45-A:528–540, 1963.
31. Mankin HJ: The reaction of articular cartilage to injury and osteoarthritis. I. *N Engl J Med* 291:1285–1292, 1974.
32. Mankin HJ: The reaction of articular cartilage to injury and osteoarthritis. II. *N Engl J Med* 291:1335–1340, 1974.
33. Maroudas A: Biophysical chemistry of cartilaginous tissues with special reference to solute and fluid transport. *Biorheology* 12:233–248, 1975.
34. Meachim G: The effect of scarification on articular cartilage in the rabbit. *J Bone Joint Surg* 45-B:150–161, 1963.
35. Mitchell N, Shepard N: The resurfacing of adult rabbit articular cartilage by multiple perforations through the subchondral bone. *J Bone Joint Surg* 58-A:230–233, 1976.
36. Otte P: Die regenerationsunfähigkeit des gelenkknorpels. *Z Orthop* 90:299–303, 1958.
37. Radin EL, Paul IL, Tolkoff MJ: Subchondral bone changes in patients with early degenerative joint disease. *Arthritis Rheum* 13:400–450, 1970.
38. Random House Inc: *The Random House Dictionary of the English Language*. New York, 1969.
39. Rodale JI: The synonym finder. Emmaus, PA, Rodale Press, Inc., 1978.
40. Roth V, Mow VC: The intrinsic tensile behavior of the matrix of bovine articular cartilage and its variation with age. *J Bone Joint Surg* 62-A:1102–1117, 1980.
41. Salter RB, Field P: The effects of continuous compression on living articular cartilage. An experimental investigation. *J Bone Joint Surg* 42-A:31–49, 1960.
42. Salter RB, Simmonds DF, Malcolm BW, et al: The biological effect of continuous passive motion on the healing of full-thickness defects in articular cartilage. *J Bone Joint Surg* 62-A:1232–1251, 1980.
43. Thaxter TH, Mann RA, Anderson CE: Degeneration of immobilized knee joints in rats. Histological and autoradiographic study. *J Bone Joint Surg* 47-A:567–585, 1965.
44. Urist MR: Recent advances in physiology of calcification. *J Bone Joint Surg* 46-A:889–900, 1964.
45. Wigren A, Falk J, Wik O: The healing of cartilage injuries under the influence of joint immobilization and repeated hyaluronic acid injections. *Acta Orthop Scand* 49:121–133, 1978.

# CHAPTER SIX

# Panel Discussion: Does Chondromalacia Patella Exist?

MODERATOR, ERIC L. RADIN, M.D.

Let's start off by asking questions of individual members of the panel, but if any of you have anything else you want to add, please raise your hand and I will be glad to call on you. Dr. Meachim, could you define chondromalacia pathologically please?

**Dr. Meachim:** "I don't think one can define chondromalacia pathologically except in the literal sense meaning a softening of cartilage. It seems to me that beyond that the pathologist becomes baffled by the nomenclature that is used by the orthopedic surgeon."

**Moderator:** "All right, can I summarize it by saying that it is just soft cartilage?"

**Dr. Meachim:** "Indeed so, and I think the first thing we do not know is the etiology of the softening phenomenon. I feel the honest answer to this question as a histologist is simply to say that it is a descriptive term without any clinical significance to it whatsoever."

**Moderator:** "All right, the next question is, what is the clinical definition of chondromalacia? For that we want to call on several of our panel. The most puzzled looking one and the most shocked one is Mr. Goodfellow but Carroll Laurin has his hand up."

**Dr. Laurin:** "Chondromalacia is like sciatica, pain down the leg. It is a symptom complex, herniated lumbar intervertebral disc disease becomes sciatica."

**Moderator:** "Mr. Goodfellow, would you like to comment?"

**Mr. Goodfellow:** "Chondromalacia is clinically defined as anterior knee pain. It is a nonspecific clinical term and doesn't really help us except to localize the difficulty to the anterior (patella femoral) compartment of the knee."

**Moderator:** "To summarize what's been said so far, is that clinically the term chondromalacia is not very helpful and that one would feel more comfortable for example calling a pain in the anterior knee 'anterior knee pain.' The reason is that calling it chondromalacia doesn't necessarily tell the surgeon what is going on. All right, let's have some other comments, Paul Maquet."

**Dr. Maquet:** "I recognize a variety of causes of pain in the anterior knee and to treat specifically, what Professor Pauwels called causative treatment, or to treat the cause, we must specifically define the cause of the anterior knee pain in each patient."

**Moderator:** "I think that the term chondromalacia used clinically is like internal derangement of the knee. That is just a corollary of what Dr. Laurin has said. Our profession has succeeded, over the past two decades, to get rid of the term internal derangement except as a term which implies you have to do something else to establish a diagnosis. The term chondromalacia should imply to us that we need to do something to establish a proper diagnosis. If the term chondromalacia, used clinically, leads us to some specific actions to establish the etiology of the pathogenesis of the clinical syndrome of anterior knee pain, then the term chondromalacia may retain some clinical usefulness. But if chondromalacia continues to be used as a wastebasket term, that is to say, that patients will continue to be signed out with that diagnosis, then the term chondromalacia is absolutely useless clinically and should be discarded."

**Dr. Casscells:** "It would seem to be that we would be better off without using the term chondromalacia at all and so I agree with you. The term chondromalacia should be reserved as a pathological description only."

**Moderator:** "So you are more comfortable with the use of the term chondromalacia as a purely pathological term; and are you comfortable by what has been suggested by the panel, that clinical chondromalacia should be thought of as an internal derangement of the anterior knee and about as meaningful diagnostically as the term sciatica."

**Dr. Casscells:** "I am not happy with that either."

**Moderator:** "You appear not to want to use the term chondromalacia at all, and what you are implying is that the topic of this symposium should have been 'The Etiology and Treatment of Pain in the Anterior Knee', would that be closer to what your beliefs are?"

**Dr. Casscells:** "Yes, using the term chondromalacia clinically blocks the diagnostic process and, therefore, an intelligent treatment. For example . . . "

**Moderator:** "We are going to talk about treatment tomorrow so I am going to cut you off with the rest of that thought. Let's just stay with the etiological problems today. Mr. Goodfellow?"

**Mr. Goodfellow:** "We seem to all agree but we are stuck with two things. The pathological description, and I don't know that that is even good pathology. Better to say the morphological description of abnormal cartilage. I think everyone will agree with that and by conviction, if you like, we are also stuck with a widely understood meaning when you talk about chondromalacia, to most people in this room, as they would feel you were describing a clinical syndrome as well. In that it is quite clear that these two things may overlap somewhat but they are very different entities. As you heard this morning it is normal for people over a certain age to have morphological changes in the patella described as chondromalacia. The other side of the coin is that there are people who have the absolutely characteristic syndrome without detectable change on the patella at all. Two comments on this: There was a paper published about 10 years ago that I don't think received the recognition it should, which came upon a number of patella removed for anterior knee pain. They examined them all pathologically and found very little change in the articular cartilage in most of the specimens but some very interesting subchondral bone changes.

Another comment is that almost everyone that has written on the subject in the last 10 years, including many people in this room, have commented that they, in a certain proportion of their cases, have found normal articular cartilage when they open the knee. George Bentley from Liverpool recently said that arthroscopically this was as high as 50%."

**Moderator:** "Do you want to comment further at this point, George Meachim?"

**Dr. Meachim:** "Only with reluctance. I am not happy about some of the terms that are being used. What do people mean by pathological? What do people mean by normal and abnormal? I think there is a tendency to think that any cartilage that doesn't exactly replicate the technicolor picture in our histology textbooks is abnormal. What we are really saying is that the cartilage is no longer in pristine condition. And surely it will be a tremendous achievement on nature's art if our cartilages were to remain in the same state, as they were initially manufactured, throughout their working life. So I would feel that a noncommital term, like age-related to generation, if you like, gets us off the hook of these rather philosophical arguments."

**Moderator:** "Excellent. Your comment brings forward about 8 or 10 other questions that the audience has sent up here."

**Dr. Meachim:** "I doubt if I know any of the answers to those questions."

**Moderator:** "The reason that all of these people came here, George, is that they assumed you did know."

**Mr. Goodfellow:** "George Meachim doesn't want us to use the term chondromalacia at all but rather talk about age-related changes. Maybe we would be better off not using the term chondromalacia ever."

**Moderator:** "We seem to be moving in an interesting direction which I hope is clear. Just to summarize the way the panel is beginning to move, let's take a vote, maybe we can cut down on discussion. Does the panel agree that the presence of deterioration of articular cartilage is not necessarily the cause of any symptoms, how many would agree to that?"

**Mr. Goodfellow:** "There is no room for democracy in science."

**Moderator:** "In answer to that I must quote a comment in a letter I received from John Goodfellow agreeing to participate in this course. He said in that letter that this symposium would probably be more theology than science and, of course, his premonition turned out to be true. Was there general agreement over there among the panel? Yes, apparently there is. O.K., so that is the first step. The second that I want you to talk about is the source of the cartilage lesions. Let's start with this. George Meachim described deep and superficial cartilage lesions. Therefore, the initiation of cartilage change occurs in both the surface and the deep layers. Do you feel there is any difference in the tendency to progress of these two kinds of lesions?"

Does everyone in the audience understand what we are talking about? George Meachim's talk and later John Goodfellow said that cartilage lesions do not necessarily have to initiate at the surface. The standard fibrillation we are all familiar with does, but some of the lesions described don't. They begin deep down below the surface, just above the tidemark which represents the transition from articular cartilage to calcified cartilage. Weakened by these deep horizontal fissures an attack on the surface could obviously occur. So the question raised by a number in the audience is, do you think there is any difference clinically between these lesions? George Meachim, you have probably seen more of them than any of us."

**Dr. Meachim:** "I have seen a lot of them in the necropsy room but, of course, the problem is one doesn't know what significance they have had. I think what surprised me when looking at cartilage lesions histologically and with India ink is the wide variety of morphological changes that can occur in addition to the four we have mentioned already this morning: shearing, abrasion, fibrillation, and fasciculation. There are at least another four or five one could mention. Quite often these occur together at the same site, therefore I think it is difficult to theorize about their prospective potential with this exception. Once abrasive wear is occurring I think it has a strong potential to progress down to bone exposure."

**Moderator:** "Have you seen this sort of lesion occurring both on the medial and lateral facets of the patella?"

**Dr. Meachim:** "We have had one example of abrasive wear on the medial facet that I can recall."

**Moderator:** "But what you are implying is that progressive lesions mostly occur laterally."

**Dr. Meachim:** "Indeed, sir, yes."

**Moderator:** "All right, let me ask John Goodfellow to comment next since he has also described these deep horizontal lesions both this morning and in the *Journal of Bone and Joint Surgery*."

**Mr. Goodfellow:** "The characteristic lesions which we have described on the odd facet have no distinct symptomatic difference with other cartilage lesions."

**Moderator:** "Do you think they might be separate lesions?"

**Mr. Goodfellow:** "Yes."

**Moderator:** "Well then, the next obvious question, again asked by several members of the audience, is, are the cartilage deteriorations necessarily symptomatic? Dr. Meachim, being a pathologist, begs the issue saying his patient has complained very little. But the rest of us are not so well blessed. Perhaps we can get some comments from the other panelists."

**Mr. Goodfellow:** "The answer is that cartilage lesions are not necessarily symptomatic."

**Moderator:** "All right, Paul Maquet, do you agree or disagree with that?"

**Dr. Maquet:** "I agree with that."

**Moderator:** "Carroll Laurin, agree or disagree?"

**Dr. Laurin:** "What did he say?"

**Moderator:** "What he said was that deterioration of articular cartilage does not necessarily become symptomatic or regress."

**Dr. Laurin:** "I agree."

**Moderator:** "Rudolf Lemperg, he is nodding his head, he agrees. David Hungerford?"

**Dr. Hungerford:** "I think it is a little more complex than that, because I think one can certainly agree that all cartilage lesions are not always symptomatic. Subsurface lesions are not ever symptomatic and subcartilage lesions are sometimes symptomatic."

**Moderator:** "What about saying subcartilage lesions are associated with symptoms?"

**Dr. Hungerford:** "We have had the opportunity to demonstrate that subcartilage lesions are symptomatic, in other words, we have had the occasion at Johns Hopkins with some of these open under local anesthesia to apply direct pressure to the articular cartilage and then produce patient symptoms. I have done this arthroscopically as well and we have produced patient symptoms with direct pressure using the arthroscope. I think you can say that subcartilage lesions are symptomatic. If the individual on which you are applying pressure is symptomatic at that particular moment you can repeat that several times and every time you press, it gives pain in that particular circumstance in that particular patient at that particular moment."

**Moderator:** "O.K., Ward Casscells?"

**Dr. Casscells:** "I agree."

**Dr. Meachim:** "Just to support what has been said, at postmortem so many patients show degenerative changes it would statistically seem to me unlikely that every cartilage lesion is painful in every joint."

**Moderator:** "That leads us to the next question, which is, what causes anterior knee pain, Dr. Meachim?"

**Dr. Meachim:** "Only to repeat what has been said already. The possibilities you want us to consider are: a) Pain coming from the bone; and b) The possibility of what we call gunk synovitis."

**Moderator:** "Gunk synovitis? Named after Professor Gunk in Liverpool?"

**Dr. Meachim:** "No, no, named after someone in Philadelphia, GUNK. In terms of the possibility of synovial and capsulary reactions one had a number of possibilities to consider, debris coming from the cartilage, chemical products from the cartilage, even possibly immunological responses to cartilage products."

**Moderator:** "Mr. Goodfellow?"

**Mr. Goodfellow:** "Two things; one is a mechanism that George was already referring to and the other is scarification of the anterior knee cartilage. I think we should address ourselves to that."

**Moderator:** "Excellent, and that in fact is the next subject, what are the causes of anterior knee pain. Why do you panelists think patients with soft cartilage have pain?"

**Dr. Hungerford:** "I think they hurt because of the abnormal transmission of force through abnormal cartilage to either normally responsive bone or perhaps abnormally responsive bone. I think you have two phenomena that you will have to explain. One is the patient who has pain associated with high contact pressures and that is an off-on phenomenon. That is the individual who comes down an 8-inch step, has pain at the moment the knee applies a heavy load to his anterior knee and particularly to the patellofemoral joint. The more common phenomenon is the individual who has less specific and more diffuse pain either after repetitive activities or after prolonged immobilization such as sitting. I don't think that these two syndromes necessarily are synonymous, they may be but they don't have to be. The vascular side of the phenomenon needs to be looked at. Since most of the nerves of the bone are intimately associated with the vessels and we really haven't addressed that thought I think there is an increasing association in terms of burning pain which is deep, somewhat diffuse, resembling a variety of conditions, including avascular necrosis, infection, arthritis, and anterior knee pain. I think a direct pressure contact with bone causes abnormal pressures being transmitted to it, perhaps to abnormally sensitive areas to those pressures perhaps due to vascular changes in the bone. Either of these two phenomena could exist."

**Moderator:** "Just to expand on that, haven't you measured some venous pressures in the patella?"

**Dr. Hungerford:** "We have measured pressures in both the distal femur and patella. The patella is quite hard to measure because the bone is very hard and it is difficult to be sure exactly where you are. But in the ones we have measured they have been abnormally high. They have been mostly in reflex sympathetic dystrophy patients which is another phenomenon that perhaps we had better not discuss today. There is one thing though that is very interesting about the pressures and that is that if you measure the pressure in the distal femur at the time of quadriceps contraction you get a marked temporary elevation of the venous pressure and at the release of the quadriceps contraction a decrease in the venous pressure which takes several minutes to return to the base line. That is an interesting phenomenon in relationship to isometric exercises and the relief of anterior knee pain."

**Moderator:** "Any further comments about the causes of knee pain? Is everybody happy here with GUNK synovitis and bone pain as the two major causes?"

I am going to give Carroll Laurin the floor in a minute because I want him to comment on some work he has been doing on this.

**Moderator:** "Paul Maquet?"

**Dr. Maquet:** "I believe pain has something to do with pressure in the joint."

**Moderator:** "I might just add something and that is that in an experiment done several years ago, Don Chrisman took normal articular cartilage from one knee of a rabbit and injected it into the other knee which was normal at the time. What he observed was profound synovitis and he attributed that to the sulfated proteoglycans which the synovial cells didn't really appreciate at all. Although we will talk about treatment tomorrow, this would certainly be consistent with the clinical observation that sometimes just a lavage at the time of arthroscopy relieves pain and this is what we are talking about when Dr. Meachim and others speak of GUNK synovitis."

**Mr. Goodfellow:** "I was wondering about the GUNK synovitis. I am sure this is a mechanism in some but probably in only a small minority of patients with anterior knee pain. We have for some years made a practice of doing a synovial biopsy on these people and it was a very rare patient who showed any evidence of synovial inflammation at all so I can't think this can be a common explanation for pain."

**Moderator:** "Now, there is an important issue that has been raised by several of the panelists as well as many in the audience and that is a classification of anterior knee pain so let me get someone to talk about anterior knee pain and we will ask John Insall."

**Dr. Insall:** "I think you could subdivide anterior knee pain into those that invariably have an articular lesion such as in osteoarthritis and those that don't. The nonarticular causes such as malalignment syndromes are really more common. We seldom see articular lesions associated with knee pain in runners and joggers but they do complain specifically about anterior knee pain particularly in the region of the patellar tendon since the patellar tendon has nerves in it. One wonders whether some runners don't have pain in their anterior knees which is from their patellar tendons. There is a retropatellar bursa which lies between the patella tendon and anterior tibia. I have seen inflammation in this area."

**Moderator:** "Do you think that this has been described as inflammation of the fat pad by some?"

**Dr. Insall:** "I don't know but certainly this infrapatellar bursa is particularly important as a cause of postpatellectomy pain because the patella normally holds the patellar tendon away from the anterior tibia.

Patellar tendonitis is a different disease; in that the patellar tendon fibers either at the proximal or distal end are pulled. In such patients one can discern a trigger area and pinpoint the tenderness. That is different from bursitis. The bursa is behind the patellar tendon and if you see it when you do a proximal tibial osteotomy you will find it and it is lined with synovial like membranes."

**Moderator:** "Let's now get back to talking about osteoarthritis. It's been made clear that fibrillation of cartilage deterioration does not necessarily lead to osteoarthritis and everyone on the panel seems to agree to that. What is it then that makes it progress or not progress?"

**Dr. Lemperg:** "Fibrillation becomes progressive when fibrillation provokes significant increase of enzyme activity either in the cartilage or in the synovium."

**Dr. Maquet:** "Osteoarthritis would exist when there is an imbalance between the stresses on the joint and the ability of the joint tissues to withstand those stresses."

**Mr. Goodfellow:** "In other words, a relative concentration of stress."

**Dr. Laurin:** "I think the biggest change that occurs in the transmission of stress, that creates the stress concentration, is a minor degree of subluxation of the patellofemoral joint. Even a very small alteration in the position of the patella relative to the femoral groove can cause an enormous change in the contact pattern of this joint at a time when the load was probably unchanged and, therefore, enormous increase in stress. You may have a permanent malalignment or it may be a very transient malalignment. What can occur, even very briefly, could double, triple, or quadruple the contact force and be associated with giving way and or a momentary pain. If this occurs repeatedly over a long period of time, it certainly can lead to progressive deterioration of articular cartilage."

**Moderator:** "What Carroll Laurin and Paul Maquet are saying is that stress concentrations cause progression. What Rudolf Lemperg is saying is that progression follows a misuse or overuse which creates enough bad enzymes to eat away at the cartilage. Dr. Meachim, what do you say?"

**Dr. Meachim:** "I think we have gone off on two tracks here. First, we were discussing the frequency of these various things and secondly, we have got the problem of completeness in our list of causes of anterior knee pain. I would like to make two comments. We must segregate our anterior knee pain patients into three categories, probably by age. If middle aged or older and they have had malalignment syndromes when they were young or depending on the number of sporting types we see, these could be considered overuse syndromes. I think that would be different than the patient who is very old, for in that group osteoarthrosis would be most likely. The young patients fall into the clinical chondromalacia group since some of us see patients probably preferentially in different age groups, but frequency of diagnosis will be at variance. When one sees a middle aged or older patient we should ask, "Did you have any pain in the knee when you were young? No? Are you sure? No, absolutely not? It seems to start as an increased Q-angle then they tend to put more stress on one facet than on another.""

**Moderator:** "Particularly the lateral one since the patella in the valgus knee would tend to be pulled laterally."

**Dr. Meachim:** "Again, let me emphasize that I can only comment about pathological arthritis. I define that as the progressive destruction of cartilage leading to abrasive wear and other damage to the bone. There is no doubt at all that the rate and degree of progression is very dependent upon certain factors that are not totally understood. I would submit that pain can be unrelated to the radiographic signs. One of the reasons we do not yet clearly understand the inter-relationship of the variables governing the progression of cartilage destruction is that it is very difficult to measure directly stress in cartilage. The other variables, for example the one Eric Radin suggested, the variation in subchondral bone density, has also been difficult to measure. In fact, the observations we have made on the lateral part of the patella showing subarticular calcified tissue density which is harder than that on the medial part of the patella, confirm Eric Radin's observations and is clearly another factor influencing progression. In terms of biochemical change we don't know whether the synovium produces enzymes which actually affect the cartilage. There are inhibitors in the synovial fluid. I would like to say again that progression is undoubtedly related to joint fit, and this would appear to be related to an inherent difference between male and female cartilage. In fact, there is some evidence that female cartilage is not as resistant to mechanical damage as is male cartilage."

**Moderator:** "I might also suggest that there is a difference between comparison of knee usage between men and women. David Hungerford, could you show us how subluxing patella does damage to the lateral as opposed to the medial facet of the patella as it pops back in?"

**Dr. Hungerford:** "The patella can ride laterally all the way until a part of the patella comes up to a point on the femur and once it does over the side of the femoral condyle ridge, you have a dislocated patella. Dislocation is always associated with a change in direction which is always associated with change in rotation. When you walk and run and change direction, you rotate the tibia. Then if there is subluxation, you have got to change from say a 2-mm contact area to less than 1 mm of contact. Assuming the same load, you are going to have a doubling of stress since you are talking about 2 times body weight of load or perhaps even 5 times momentarily. The stress on the cartilage must be enormous."

**Moderator:** "What about the phenomenon of popping back in, don't you think that is going to bother the medial facet?"

**Dr. Hungerford:** "No, I don't think so. I don't think that is the problem."

**Moderator:** "Well, it is the medial side which takes the brunt of things as the patella pops back in and it comes back in rather rapidly too."

**Dr. Hungerford:** "Not necessarily, unless it comes back with unusual force. The patient frequently says in the history that something happened in my knee, I don't know exactly what, I had a lot of pain, I massaged it, and I felt something kind of slide back in and it felt better."

**Moderator:** "It has been well established that the worst kind of damage one can do to articular cartilage is some kind of impact blow. The greatest impact blow would be when the patella comes back into position rather than when it goes out."

**Dr. Hungerford:** "I think if the patella is slightly damaged the first time it dislocates or subluxes, the next time it would be less capable of withstanding impact and then you would get a progressive lesion of the already damaged area."

**Moderator:** "Carroll Laurin, you have seen a lot of subluxing patella, have you had a chance to note where the cartilage damage generally is geographically located in these patellas?"

**Dr. Laurin:** "On the medial patellar ridge or the medial patellar facet."

**Moderator:** "You found the damage to be more on the lateral side of the patella cartilage in chronic subluxing patterns?"

**Dr. Laurin:** "Medial."

**Moderator:** "Please explain."

**Dr. Laurin:** "In patellar malalignment, malacic lesions developed on the medial side of the patellofemoral joint. This was also the finding experimentally."

**Moderator:** "In these patients who have recurring subluxations, John Goodfellow, have you had the chance to tell whether the cartilage lesion created by this was medial or lateral?"

**Mr. Goodfellow:** "I cannot say."

**Moderator:** "Ward Casscells, you have looked at a great number of knees with your arthroscope. Have you noticed any predilection toward a lesion in chronic dislocators or chronic subluxators between the medial and lateral facets?"

**Dr. Casscells:** "The same lesions are usually lateral."

**Moderator:** "He is telling us that lesions on the medial facet tend not to progress."

**Dr. Casscells:** "But most cartilage damage I have seen occurs on the medial facet."

**Dr. Meachim:** "We seem to have uncovered a major schism here."

**Moderator:** "The problem may be one of definition or terminology. Nonprogressive damage is what I mean by fibrillation."

**Dr. Casscells:** "My experience would agree with the observation originally made but with a high association of cartilage lesions situated in exactly the same area that David Hungerford indicates in his diagram. That is just the lateral side of the upper crest. There is no doubt about that in my mind."

**Dr. Laurin:** "I think we have to separate instability and malalignment. They are not always associated. You can have a recurrent instability in the form of an associated muscular or ligamentous imbalance without the patient having an increased Q-angle and with the patella centered in all three views. And yet the patient has clearly had a major instability at some point. There are the more regular recurrent instabilities that fall into the category. The patient has a recurrent giving way and you see a subluxation at 40° of flexion with the patella coming out of its congruent channel either intermittently or perhaps repeatedly in a single place in the flexion arc every time. On the other hand, malalignment is a form of permanent dislocation. Subluxation and malalignment are not synonyms in that sense. A lesion may be a fracture of cartilage on the medial facet or it may be an incongruity which may be so great that a piece of paper can be passed between the medial cartilage, medial facet on the trochlea. That means the contact area is decreased and I have to believe that, if anything, joints transmit stress, then this has some significance. If there is any damage to the patella from malalignment it is different than the damge from chronic subluxation."

**Moderator:** "We have a great number of questions about Carroll Laurin's presentation and particularly about conditions under which the skyline view of the patella is taken. Is it 20 or 30° of flexion, Carroll?"

**Dr. Laurin:** "20°."

**Moderator:** "The next thing is, does it matter whether the quadriceps is contracted or not at the time you take the picture?"

**Dr. Laurin:** "No."

**Moderator:** "Well, some people say the position of the patella on the skyline view can be influenced by whether the quadriceps is contracted or not. Since it is impossible to stand with the knee flexed 20° and not contract the patella, one should probably ask for the muscle to be contracted. Maldague has shown that in taking a view of the quadriceps relaxed you may see the patella slide off laterally although that may not have any meaningful terms in regards to the activities of daily living.

Now the final question. Someone wants to know 'Is the softening of the articular cartilage irreversible'? Does that ever go away, Rudolf Lemperg?

**Dr. Lemperg:** "It is very unlikely fibrillation goes away."

**Moderator:** "Does anyone feel that fibrillation goes away? Well, I think everyone agrees with you, Rudolf. When fibrillation occurs, although it doesn't necessarily progress, it doesn't go away."

# CHAPTER SEVEN

# Chondromalacia Patella and Its Relationship to Anterior Femoral Pain

**S. WARD CASSCELLS, M.D.**

The first part of this presentation will be a discussion of the epidemiology of a condition which, in this meeting, we have referred to as anterior knee pain. Inasmuch as the material I am going to show comes from a cadaver study, I am afraid that the term anterior knee pain is inappropriate, and I will have to refer to it by that undesirable name, chondromalacia.

Those who have read the literature on this subject over the past many years must have come to the conclusion that chondromalacia of the patella is inevitable by the time someone reaches 40 or 50 years of age, and from then on, it is progressive with increasing pain and disability. The basis for this opinion is mostly anecdotal, though there are several reports (5, 9) which appeared in the German literature many years ago which are supportive of this belief. The data I am about to present derived from a cadaver study I carried out some years ago (1).

It was very fortunate that throughout the 6-year period during which this study took place that it represented the older age group, the average age being 70. Only 8% of these 369 knees were in individuals below the age of 50. Thus, we had a very good idea of what the knee joint looked like at the end of a normal life span.

In this group of cadaver knees, there were 37% (Fig. 7.1) in which the patellar surface was grossly normal. In 25% (Fig. 7.2), there was very minor damage, less than 1 cm in diameter, with only the superficial layers of the cartilage involved. This was arbitrarily classified as a Grade I lesion. In 27% (Fig. 7.3), a Grade II lesion was present which was defined as 1–2 cm in diameter

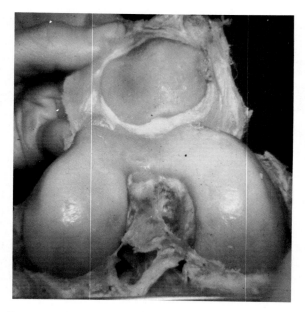

**Figure 7.1.** Essentially normal joint surfaces in a 74-year old man. There is very minor damage to the articular surface of the patella in the region of the odd facet.

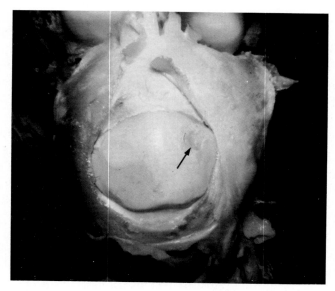

**Figure 7.2.** Small superficial Grade I type lesion involving the medial facet of the patella.

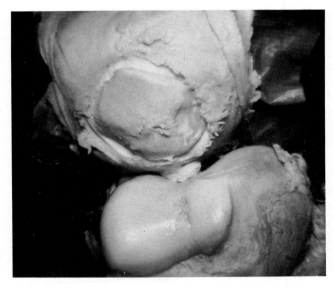

**Figure 7.3.**   Grade II lesion of the patella and femur with involvement of the deeper layers of the cartilage.

with some of the deeper layers of the cartilage involved, but bone was not exposed. Based on clinical experience, it is doubtful that Grade I or even Grade II lesions were even symptomatic. Grade III lesions (Fig. 7.4) were present in 6% of the cases and signified a defect 2–4 cm in diameter in which some bone was exposed. Grade IV lesions 5% were anything larger than this and included those lesions in which the patella was entirely denuded of articular cartilage. Thus, there were only 11% of these 369 knees which were of undoubted clinical significance.

These patellar lesions were not only graded as to severity, but were also located on the patellar surface. This is a rather controversial subject with little agreement as to where the lesions commence, whether they progress, and how rapidly. There does seem to be universal agreement, however, that the lesions of the extreme medial pole of the patella are of little clinical significance and probably do not progress. This area of the patella has been referred to as the odd facet (Fig. 7.5). In some patellae, this is a well-developed structure, in others, it is poorly developed and scarcely qualifies for this designation of

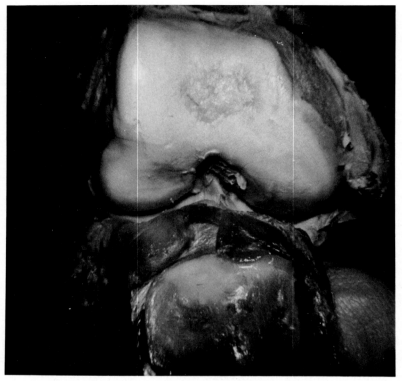

**Figure 7.4.** A 3-cm lesion of the femur with involvement of most of the articular cartilage.

odd facet. The etiology of a lesion in this area is not known. I have seen it occur following patellar dislocation. However, in most cases, when it is present, where is no such history of dislocation. Goodfellow (4) has stated that it is perhaps the result of nonuse. It articulates with the femur only in full flexion.

In this groups of cadavers, the lesions were confined to the medial facet of the patella in 25% with no effort being made to differentiate between the medial facet and the so-called odd facet. In 12%, the lesion was located on the central ridge of the patella dividing the medial from the lateral facet, and in another 12%, the lesion was confined to the lateral facet. In 51%, it was generalized, and there was no way of knowing where the lesion started. There was nothing in this study that supported Outerbridge's theory that the lesion invariably commences on

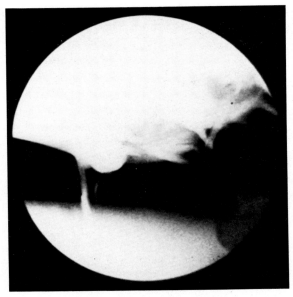

**Figure 7.5.**   A somewhat magnified veiw of chondromalacia of the odd facet of the patella seen arthroscopically. A similar lesion seen in Figure 7.1.

the medial facet due to a ridge on the adjacent femoral condyle, a so-called "Outerbridge Ridge" (8).

In the course of this cadaver study, measurements were also made of the heights of the femoral condyles and the depth of the intervening groove or sulcus. The lateral condyle averaged 4.5 mm higher than the medial with extremes being from 0–10 mm (Fig. 7.6). The average depth of the sulcus was 5.2 mm, again with a wide range from a depth of 1–10 mm (Fig. 7.7) and a flat dysplastic femur with no sulcus at the other extreme. It was hoped that by these measurements, it might be possible to establish a cause-and-effect relationship and a possible etiological factor in the development of chondromalacia. There were so many variables, including the location and severity of the patellar lesions and the varying heights of the condyles and depths of the sulcus that it was not possible to draw any inferences. It is, of course, recognized that a flat dysplastic anterior femoral surface permits the patella to slide laterally and dislocate, and this, of course, is a well-recognized cause of damage of the patellar articular surface.

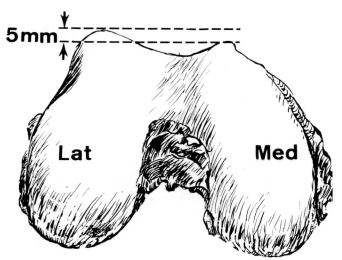

**Figure 7.6.** A drawing showing the height and configuration of the condyles in the average femur.

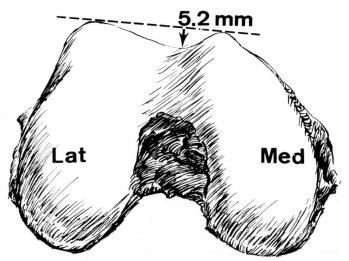

**Figure 7.7.** Depth and configuration of the sulcus in the anterior femur of the average specimen.

In general, the incidence of these patellar lesions was roughly similar to that found in a study of Chinese knees by Marrar and Pillay (7). Some additional information was obtained from this study which did not lend itself to any definite conclusions.

Lesions of the patellofemoral area were found on both sides of the joint in some patients, but they were also found on one side of the joint or the other in many others, the patellar side being considerably more frequent. These lesions also varied considerably in their physical characteristics. Those on the medial facet seemed to be better localized with more vertical edges, and somehow gave the appearance of being more stable (Fig. 7.7). This certainly was suggested, when these minor lesions of Grade I and II were found in patients in the 7th and 8th decades. On the lateral side, the lesions were usually larger with beveled edges and gave the distinctive impression of being of long duration and due to excessive lateral pressure (Fig. 7.8) like

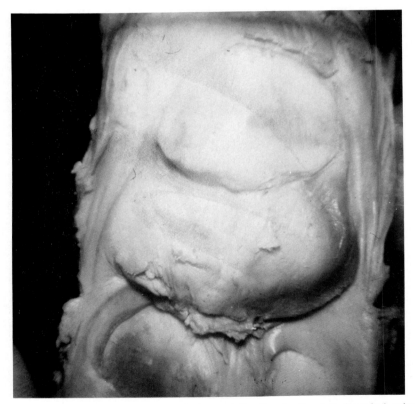

**Figure 7.8.** On the lateral side of the patella, the lesion has beveled edges suggestive of long duration.

those described by Ficat and Hungerford (3). This variation in the morphology of these lesions is seen more dramatically through the arthroscope where the surfaces (Fig. 7.9) have not been subjected to preservative solutions, as in the case of the cadavers.

Of more importance than the lesions themselves is the clinical significance, especially regarding pain. It is commonly supposed that chondromalacia is painful, and often, the term is used synonymously with anterior knee pain. Sikorski et al. (10), in the *British Journal of Bone and Joint Surgery* has gone as far as to theorize that perhaps there are two types of chondromalacia, one in which a lesion is present, and one in which there is no

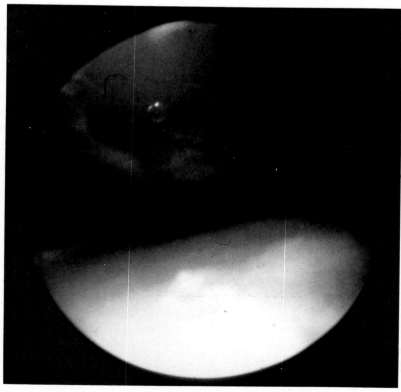

**Figure 7.9.**   Arthroscopic appearance of a lateral lesion.

lesion, both of which are painful. I am unaware of any documentation in the literature to support the belief that chondromalacia, especially in its early stages, is a painful condition. Pain in and about the knee, especially in the young, does exist in the absence of any demonstrable intra-articular pathology such as the lesions we call chondromalacia.

Since the advent of the arthroscope, clinicians have shown an increasing interest in the diagnosis and treatment of chondromalacia of the patella and anterior knee pain. In the minds of some surgeons, the two terms are synonymous. The interest generated by the development of a motorized shaver has been even more spectacular. Understandably, older clinicians who do not use the arthroscope and feel it is somewhat superfluous exhibit far less enthusiasm for the diagnostic potential of the arthroscope and the therapeutic benefits of the shaver. Before 10 years ago, there was relatively little interest in chondromalacia on the part of most clinicians. Shaving these lesions with a knife was not very successful and surgeons performing a meniscectomy paid little attention to the patella even when there was a lesion present. In like manner, pediatricians who saw young patients in their office with vague knee pains tended to dismiss them with the diagnosis of growing pains and ensured the patients that the pain would disappear. Usually it did.

When I analyzed my first 1000 arthroscopic cases (2), there were 160 in which there was pain in the knee but no intra-articular explanation. In an effort to better understand this relationship between the pain and chondromalacia, a series of 106 consecutive knees were reviewed which had been arthroscoped. In all of these knees, there was either pain, chondromalacia, or both. In 33%, there was chondromalacia but no pain. In 45%, there was pain but no chondromalacia, and in 22%, there were both pain and chondromalacia. Patients with chondromalacia of the patella may or may not have crepitus, depending on the location of the lesion and the severity. My studies in this regard have led me to believe that true patellar crepitus is pathognomonic of chondromalacia but not all patients with chondromalacia have crepitus. There are, of course, pops and clicks which emanate from the patellofemoral joint on motion, but these should not be referred to as crepitus. Following this review, all patients who came into my office for whatever reason were checked for crepitus and not infrequently it was found in patients who had no knee complaints whatsoever. The arthroscope is the most accurate method of making this diagnosis whether it is a surface lesion as it usually is or whether there is a softened but intact deeper lesion which can be diagnosed by probing.

The question of whether or not making an accurate diagnosis is of any value to the patient depends upon what you are prepared to do if you find a lesion on the patella. Almost all arthroscopists treat these lesions with the motorized shaver without knowing whether or not any long-term beneficial effects will result from this procedure. The appearance of the lesion certainly can be improved and removing the damaged tissue may reduce the amount of lysosomal enzymes which are released into the joint, and, thus, have a stabilizing effect on the lesion. All the damaged articular cartilage cannot be removed with the shaver and no one with any knowledge or experience in dealing with damaged articular cartilage believes that these defects will heal. It is fairly safe to say that no harm will result from treating these lesions in this fashion.

In the matter of treatment of these knees, the question arises as to whether we are treating a pathological condition which was described at least 75 years ago and later named chondromalacia or are we treating a symptom complex, a painful knee, which for the lack of a better term is called chondromalacia even when no lesion of the patellar surface is present? Very few patients would agree to have surgery on their knee solely because of the crepitus, and probably, the majority of physicians would not suggest it. On the other hand, patients with painful knees do come seeking treatment and the arthroscope is of very little value in the diagnosis and treatment of patients with idiopathic or anterior knee pain. In my experience (2), most of these young patients do not have chondromalacia and as Ficat and Hungerford (3) have said, anterior knee pain should not be considered synonymous with chondromalacia. Some of these patients with knee pain do have a tight lateral capsule with lateral tracking of the patella though many in my experience have essentially normal patellar tracking. Although malalignment of the patella and lateral patellar tracking can be diagnosed with the arthroscope. it usually can be diagnosed clinically by inspection, palpation, and by appropriate tangential x-rays. However, if the clinician believes that lateral retinacular release is indicated, then a thorough evaluation of the joint by the arthroscope is indicated. This is especially true when the possibility of a meniscal tear is suspected. Numerous surgical procedures have been devised to relieve this pain which not infrequently are unsuccessful. Lateral release falls in this category, as does the Maquet Procedure and proximal realignment. Unfortunately, there are not always clear-cut guidelines as to which, if any, of these procedures should be carried out to relieve the patient's pain.

Arthroscopy, then, has a somewhat limited role in the diagnosis and treatment of conditions of the patellofemoral area. There is a tendency to overuse and sometimes abuse new diagnostic tests and technical advances in surgery and this is true of arthroscopy. Although little or no harm to the patients results, it is a very expensive means of making a diagnosis and for that reason if for no other, it should be used judiciously.

The etiology of this pathological condition has not been addressed at this meeting. It is my own view that trauma and mechanical factors are certainly the main cause. I do not believe that aging per se is very important. Although it is a common disease, it is not a universal disease, and the incidence of advanced changes at age 70 was only 11% in the study I carried out. Articular cartilage does withstand the rigors of a normal lifespan in the absence of trauma and malalignment and infrequently undergoes progressive degradation. I believe that chondromalacia is overdiagnosed and overtreated. When you consider some surgical solution for this condition, I think we might remember the admonition that has been attributed to Jack Hughston (6), "there is no orthopaedic condition that cannot be made worse by surgery."

**References**

1. Casscells SW: Gross pathological changes in the knee joint of the aged individual—A study of 300 cases. *Clin Orthop* 132:225–232, 1978.
2. Casscells SW: The place of arthroscopy in the diagnosis and treatment of internal derangement of the knee and analysis of 1000 cases. *Clin Orthop*

3. Ficat RP, Hungerford DS: *Disorders of the Patello-Femoral Joint.* Baltimore, Williams & Wilkins, 1977, pp. 172–174.
4. Goodfellow J, Hungerford DS, Woods C, et al: Patello-femoral joint mechanics and pathology chondromalacia patella. *J Bone Joint Surg* 58B:291–299, 1976.
5. Heine J: Arthritis deformans. *Arch Pathol Anat* 260:521, 1926.
6. Hughston J: Personal communication.
7. Marrar BD, Pillay VK: Chondromalacia of the patella in Chinese, a postmortem study. *J Bone Joint Surg* 57A:342–345, 1975.
8. Outerbridge RE: Further studies in etiology of chondromalacia of the patella. *J Bone Joint Surg* 46B:179, 1974.
9. Owre A: Chondromalacia of the patellae. *Acta Chir Scand* 77:(Suppl)41, 1936.
10. Sikorski JM, Peters J, Watt I: The importance of femoral rotation in chondromalacia patellae as shown by serial radiography. *J Bone Joint* Surg 61B:435, 1979.

# CHAPTER EIGHT

# Lateral Fascia Release and Lateral Hyperpressure Syndrome

**PAUL FICAT, M.D.**

The causes of disorders (2) of articular cartilage are the same as those of degenerative joint disease since usually the chondropathies form the initial stage of a more advanced disorder which involves all the components of the joint. The three main etiological factors are trauma, structural disorders, and mechanical problems, such as dysplasia, patellar instability, and joint overload. It is this last category that I wish to discuss.

The patellofemoral joint is the most unstable of all joints, and the most prone to dysplasia, but, thanks to the thickness of its articular cartilage, it also has the greatest capacity for functional adaptation. Biomechanically, the patella is in dynamic equilibrium under the permanent control of two restraining mechanisms which cross each other a right angles and exist even in the embryo of 40 mm. The transverse restraint consists of the medial and lateral patellar retinacula reinforced by the corresponding vastus muscles. The longitudinal restraint is formed by the patellar tendon inferiorly and the quadriceps tendon superiorly. With the leg fully extended, these two structures form an angle of more than 170° with the apex at the patella. This angle is the result of the anatomical valgus of the knee. This valgus angle, together with the physiological "Q"-angle of the patellar tendon, leads to a phenomenon which we have called the "law of valgus" and which explains the predominance of lateral instability in displacements of the patella and the predominance of lateral compartment involvement in patellofemoral pathology. This valgus tendency is counteracted: 1) by the angle of inclination of the lateral facet of the trochlea which extends further upward and forward than the medial facet; 2) by the resistance of the medial retinaculum;

or 3) by the contraction of the horizontal, inferior component of vastus medialis. Finally, the resultant of the forces of flexion pulls the patella into the trochlear groove. This resultant increases with increasing flexion and reaches 3.3 times body weight in descending stairs. Abnormalities of the distribution of forces around the knee can lead to instability or excessive pressure on the joint surfaces and morphological anomalies or dysplasias may mean that the surfaces are incongruous with consequent overload and instability. In 3000 arthrograms done for internal derangement of the knee, we found evidence of chondropathy in 61% and the site involved was: lateral compartment in 55%, central zone in 30%, medial compartment in 15%. In other words, the syndrome of excessive lateral pressure is the most common form of this disorder (5).

From the point of view of etiology, the syndrome has two related causes: the first consists of an imbalance of the patellar retinacula, with the lateral predominating. This may be due to excessive tension laterally with hypertrophy and sclerosis of the lateral patellofemoral soft tissues. There may be associated hypertrophy of the vastus lateralis or lateral obliquity of the patellar tendon, that is, an increase in the Q-angle. But the syndrome of excessive lateral pressure is paradoxically more common in genu varum than in genu valgum. Alternatively, the imbalance may be due to a deficiency of the medial soft tissues, particularly vastus medialis. Lateral instability may be recurrent, as with recurrent subluxation or dislocation of the patella, or may be associated with a rotatory instability of the knee. The second cause of the syndrome is bone dysplasia, of which there are two common types. The first consists of internal torsion of the femur, which projects the lateral border of the trochlea forwards and so produces a "squinting patella" and augments the pressure on the lateral compartment during flexion. This torsion may be isolated or may be associated with external tibial torsion, genu varum (the triad of Judet), or femoral anteversion. The second type of bony anomaly is a protrusion of the lateral femur, most often localized to the junction of the lateral condyle and trochlea at the meniscal impression. More rarely, one sees a protrusion of the lateral facet of the patella (a "globular" deformity of the patella).

## PATHOGENESIS OF THE PAIN

Pain can be explained by several factors:

1. Mechanical factor: alteration of the cartilage which cannot absorb the pressure in a normal way, nerves and vessels of the subchondral bone react to this stress. Hungerford demonstrated this mechanism by applying pressure on softened cartilage in a patient under local anesthesia.

2. Chemical factor: release of enzymes in the joint cavity which stimulates the nerves in the synovium.

3. Hemodynamic factor: this process is much less known. The normal pressure in bone around the knee is about 20 mm Hg.

In chondromalacia we may find an increase of bone narrow pressure in the patella, the femur, and the tibia. More often, the intramedullar pressure in the tibia is normal and the increase of the pressure is observed in the patella and the femur, i.e., in the patellofemoral joint. Sometimes, only the patella is involved (Figs. 8.1 and 8.2). After measuring the bone marrow pressure we can inject a contrast medium through the same needle to

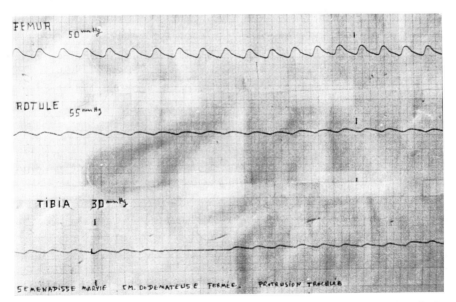

**Figure 8.1.**  Simultaneous recording of intramedullary pressure in chondromalacia of the patella. Normal rate in the metaphysis of the tibia, elevated in both sides of the patello-femoral joint.

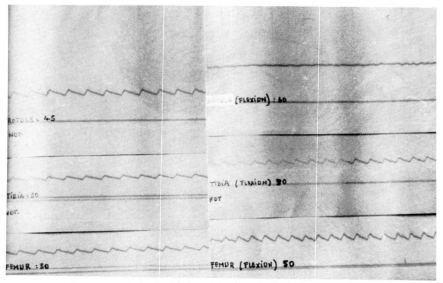

**Figure 8.2.** Intramedullary pressure, increased only in the patella but its rate increases with the passive flexion in the three bones of the knee.

determine the venous drainage. Normally all the dye is cleared up after 5 minutes. In chondromalacia, we observe a stasis in the bone marrow and a diaphyseal reflux in the femur (Fig. 8.3).

## DIAGNOSIS

All of these conditions produce a common clinical picture, the "Patellar Syndrome", which is essentially subjective and consists mainly of anterior knee pain sometimes with crepitus, locking, swelling, and giving way. Its only objective proof is provided by the axial x-ray.

### 1. Plain Skyline Views at 30°, 60°, and 90° of Flexion (Fig. 8.4)

The fundamental radiographic sign of arthrosis is narrowing of the joint line. This may be localized to the lateral compartment when the medial stabilizing structures do not counteract the tendency of the patella to tilt. The joint line is asymmetrical, being narrow laterally and opening up medially. The narrowing may be localized to the paramedian or central parts of the lateral compartment or may involve the whole of it.

The least degree of narrowing indicates a significant change in the articular cartilage, a fact that is not sufficiently well recognized. The onset of arthrosis is frequently only the terminal stage of chondrosis. Narrowing of the joint line may range from a localized diminution to complete disappearance with contact between the opposing bony surfaces.

There are three bony reactions to arthrosis. They are osteophyte formation along the lateral margin of the patella, which then curves around the edge of the trochlea (Figs. 8.5 and 8.6); thickening of the subchondral bone with increased density

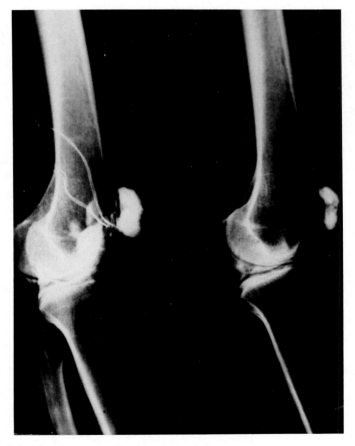

**Figure 8.3.** Phlebogram of the patella with bad drainage and stasis 30 minutes after injection.

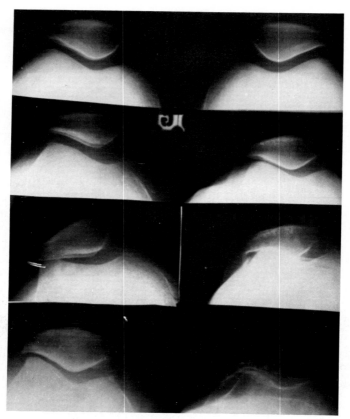

**Figure 8.4.** Diagram of narrowing of the joint line on the lateral compartment in lateral hyperpressure syndrome. *Top left:* slight narrowing compared to the opposite side. *Bottom right:* arthrosis at the terminal stage.

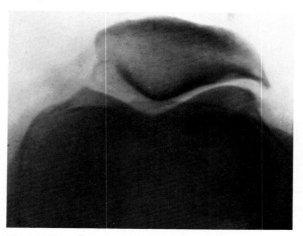

**Figure 8.5.** Typical lateral hyperpressure syndrome.

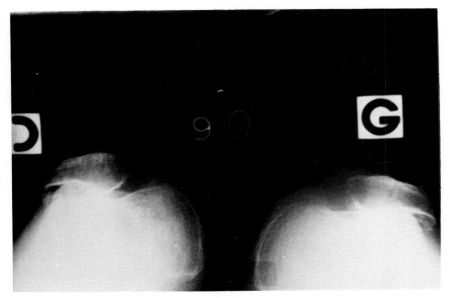

**Figure 8.6.** Eburnation of the lateral facets: it is not a permanent lateral subluxation but a lateral hyperpressure syndrome with completely destroyed cartilage.

of the underlying trabeculae and subchondral cyst formation. Secondary changes include a reorientation of the trabecular pattern toward the lateral facet and relative demineralization of the medial compartment. It is also true that one may find the same lesions on the trochlear cartilage as on the patella, both on plain radiographs and on arthrography. However, the changes are less frequent on the trochlea.

## 2. Axial Arthrograms at 30°, 45°, 60°, and 90° of Flexion

In the initial phase of chondrosis, the abnormality is confined to the cartilage and the joint line appears normal on the plain skyline view. There are no osteophytes but one may sometimes see early changes in the trabecular pattern and increased density or even subchondral cysts, which are an indirect testimony to the functional insufficiency of the articular cartilage. It is important to realize that even though the joint line is normal on plain x-rays the changes in the articular cartilage can range from softening with an intact surface to complete destruction and it is, therefore, very important to obtain contrast axial views (Fig. 8.7).

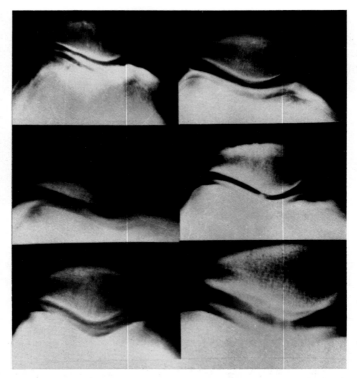

**Figure 8.7.** Diagram of axial arthrograms. *Top left:* narrowing of the central part of the lateral facet. *Top right:* slight narrowing of the critical zone (lateral paramedian zone). *Middle left:* fissure of the critical zone. *Middle right:* fissure of the critical zone. *Bottom left:* ulceration of the trochlear facet on the lateral side in front of the subchondral cyst. *Bottom right:* comblike picture of the fissuring of the critical zone.

The earliest change that may be seen is localized flattening of the articular cartilage of the patella in the "critical zone", that is, just lateral to the median ridge, or at the lateral margin of the patella. The flattening is the result of pressure applied to an area of softened cartilage. The softening can be of varying degrees of severity, from a simple loss of elasticity to complete and extensive loss of resistance which can be easily appreciated by applying digital pressure. When the softening is more advanced, the flattening extends over the whole of the lateral facet. However, in all these cases, the surface is intact and smooth and the chondromalacia is therefore "closed" (Figs. 8.8 and 8.9).

The next more severe change consists of single or multiple fissures running into the substance of the cartilage; they may be present in a zone of flattened cartilage or where the height is still normal. They may be superficial or deep and may reach down to the subchondral bone (Figs. 8.10 and 8.11). The most severe change is ulceration where there is loss of cartilage and a surface depression of variable depth, sometimes reaching down to bone (Fig. 8.12).

## ANATOMICO-PATHOLOGICAL EVOLUTION OF CHONDROMALACIA

The arthrographic changes in chondrosis and the radiographic findings in arthrosis of increasing severity allow us to reconstruct the natural history of the syndrome of excessive lateral pressure, from its origin to established arthrosis with reciprocal deformity of the patella and trochlea. Experience shows that 10 years may elapse between successive stages of the condition.

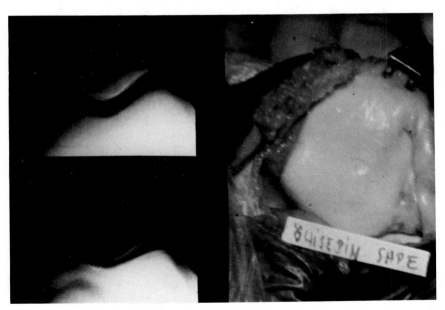

**Figure 8.8.**  Edematous chondromalacia at Stage I. *Top left:* normal joint space in the plain skyline view. *Bottom left:* narrowing of the patellar cartilage in the critical zone. *Bottom right:* photograph of the patella with softening of the lateral facet.

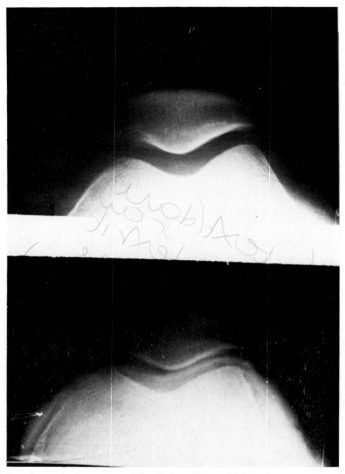

**Figure 8.9.** Contrast between plain skyline view which looks normal and the axial arthrogram which shows an important narrowing of the patellar cartilage on the lateral facet.

Macroscopically, the onset is marked by the appearance of a softened nodule of cartilage in the so-called critical zone, which is the zone of maximal pressure. At operation this can be detected with a blunt instrument. One can define an area of softening which usually is raised above the surrounding surface. The entire surface is intact and is designated as "closed" chondromalacia. This will extend slowly in both depth and breadth until the surface splits, when it becomes "open" chondromalacia. This, in turn, slowly evolves toward loss of cartilage substance and finally complete wearing away of the cartilage and eburnation of the bone. We do not believe that this sequence is inevitable. The situation can stabilize at any stage. These self-limiting lesions are often clinically silent and it is important to note that there is little correlation between the severity of the cartilage changes and the symptoms.

We have had the opportunity to biopsy cartilage from all

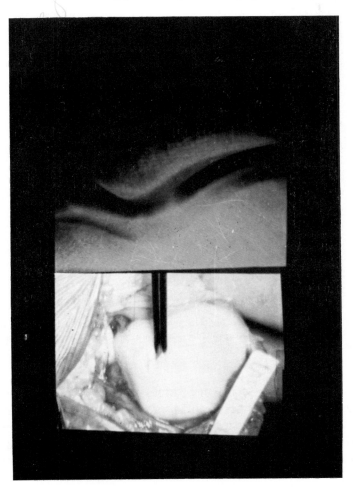

**Figure 8.10.** Fissure of the critical zone with the corresponding photograph.

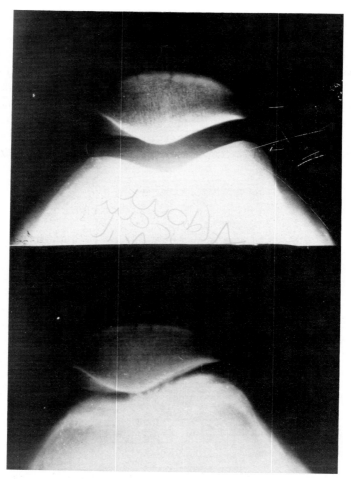

**Figure 8.11.** Contrast between a normal plain skyline view and the axial arthrogram which shows a narrowing of a softened cartilage on the lateral facet of the patella with comblike fissuration.

degrees of involvement for examination under both the optical and electron microscopes. It is possible to distinguish three phases in the evolution of the disease (4). Microscopically, the initial phase represents a reaction of the articular cartilage to the excessive pressure, a reaction which involves all three components of the cartilage. There is edema of the surface with an excess of water and a diminution in proteoglycan matrix. These changes explain the softening. There is also a breakdown in the organization of the fibrous architecture with marked variation in the diameter of individual collagen fibers, sharp angulation of some fibers, and fragmentation and disassociation of fibers, which explains the bulging of the cartilage surface. The chondrocytes show evidence of increased metabolic and secretory activity, namely, increase in the number of villi, an excess of glycogen, marked development of the Goldi apparatus, a halo of proteoglycan in the territorial matrix and evidence of cellular proliferation with the formation of pairs and clusters.

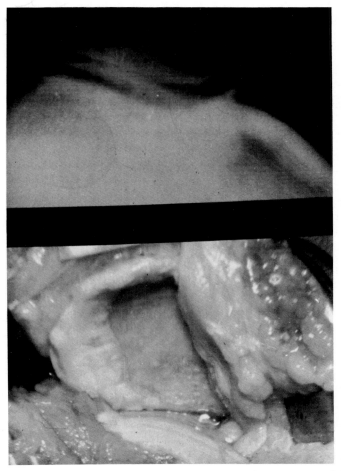

**Figure 8.12.**    Axial arthrogram shows an ulceration of the central part of the lateral facet in spite of a normal plain skyline view; corresponding photograph.

The second phase is degenerative and affects mainly the chondrocytes. There is an excess of fine filaments in the cytoplasm, dilatation of the endoplasmic reticulum, changes in the mitochondria, and the appearance of lysosomal or lipid vacuoles. In the later stages, one sees disappearance of the organelles with a tendency toward homogenization and alteration of the nucleus. The fibers tend to lose their striations and become fragmented and the disassociation is more marked. The edema between the fibers is more obvious than in the reactive stage and fissures, both superficial and deep, appear. In the third or necrotic and destructive phase, there is complete disintegration of the cytoplasm, pyknosis, and fragmentation of the nucleus and enzymatic lysis of the fibers. This is the stage of chondrocyte necrosis which leads to mechanical weakening of the cartilage, loss of substance, and the eventual involvement of the entire joint in the degenerative process.

At first, these changes are seen in the superficial part of the C2 level and then progress peripherally and to the deeper layers (C3). The reactive proliferative phases of the disease seem to last for a long time, perhaps even for years. We have found both reactive and proliferative changes in advanced open chondromalacia with edema and fissures. It seems, therefore, that necrosis of the cellular elements of cartilage is a late phenomenon which remains localized to the zone of excessive pressure, so confirming the focal nature of the mechanical arthroses. The succession of these two phases seems to correlate perfectly with the two biochemical stages of arthrosis described by Mankin, with the line of irreversibility being defined as a failure of the repair mechanism.

Turning our attention to the treatment of the syndrome of excessive lateral pressure, we see that first and foremost there is medical, conservative management. This consists of isometric quadriceps excercises, resisted flexion exercises, to develop the antagonist hamstrings, aspirin and nonsteroid anti-inflammatory drugs, and other suitable forms of physical therapy. Of our patients, 50% treated in this way avoid surgical intervention. Failure to respond to medical treatment leads to surgical intervention which is of two types. In the first place, there is surgical treatment that is directed toward changing the biomechanics of the patellofemoral joint. Second, there are measures which deal directly with the damaged cartilage. Force is applied to the patellofemoral joint in two directions. It is the lateral force, in the frontal plane that is directly responsible for the syndrome of excessive lateral pressure.

Lateral patellar release aims to decrease the valgus vector by resecting the lateral retinaculum from the level of the insertion of vastus lateralis to the tibial tubercle. This is the fundamental procedure in the treatment of the syndrome and its ideal indication includes three criteria (Figs. 8.13 and 8.14): 1) a true lateral pressure syndrome, 2) which is due to excessive tension in the lateral retinaculum, 3) and closed chondromalacia at stage I. If the syndrome is associated with instability of the patella, we can supplement the lateral release by advancement of the vastus medialis, plication of the medial capsule, or medial transposition of the tibial tubercle. If the lesion of the articular cartilage crosses the median ridge, with excessive central as well as lateral pressure, we supplement the lateral release by anterior advancement of the tibial tubercle as described by Bandi (1) and Maquet (7).

The second type of surgical treatment attacks the cartilage lesion itself. In general, where the lesion consists of softening alone and the surface is intact, only decompression is carried out. However, if fissures are present or there is loss of cartilage, there are two possible procedures. For superficial fissures, chon-

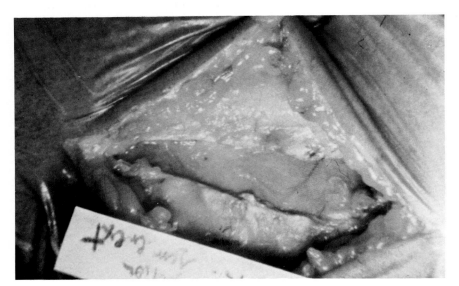

**Figure 8.13.**  Section of the thickened lateral retinaculum.

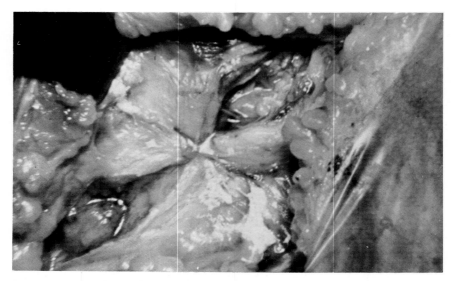

**Figure 8.14.**   Stitch with flexion of the knee to show the tension of the retinaculum.

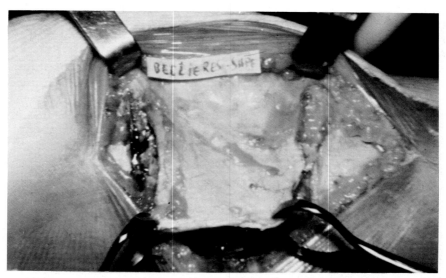

**Figure 8.15.**   Flap of the lateral retinaculum pediculated on the lateral border of the patella.

drectomy or shaving is performed to remove those fragments that would be shed into the joint. For deep fissures there are two possible procedures: 1) if the cartilage is of normal height and has a firm and elastic consistency, we drill each fissure in the manner of Pridie, 2) if the cartilage is soft and has lost its functional properties, we excise it down to bone and remove the entire subchondral plate so as to expose vascular cancellous bone, a procedure we refer to as decortication or spongialization (3). If the whole of the lateral facet is decorticated, it can be left bare or covered with a flap of retinaculum based on the edge of the patella (a patelloplasty) (Figs. 8.15 and 8.16). The same procedure is used in arthrosis of the lateral patello-femoral compartment with eburnation of both surfaces, and in this situation, the decortication of the patella is combined with drilling of the trochlea so as to maintain congruity of the joint.

## RESULTS

### Lateral Patellar Release

In a series of 144 cases with a minimum 5 years of follow-up, there were 80% good or excellent results and 20% fair or poor results. At 3 years in a series of 329 cases, there were 83.5% good results but where the indications were ideal, that is, closed chondromalacia and excessive tension in the lateral ligament, this percentage was 90%. There were three common reasons for failure of the procedure.

1. The type of lesion: major cartilage involvement extending

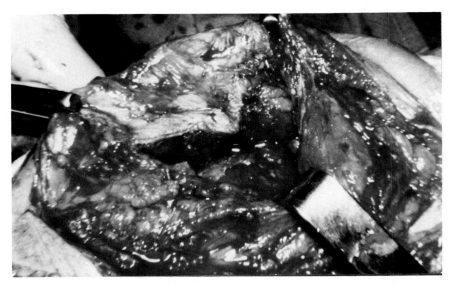

**Figure 8.16.** Resurfacing of the spongialized surface with the flap reflected on the patella.

either widely over the surface or deeply in one area. Vivalta et al. (8) found that the number of good and excellent results were 12% lower in this group also post-traumatic lesions with chondrocyte necrosis and chondrosclerosis, which seems to be irreversible.

2. Inadequate surgical decompression: this is particularly liable to happen when there is involvement of more than the lateral facet or when there is underlying dysplasia or rotational deformity.

3. Excessive decompression: produces a medial tilt of the patella with secondary medial chondromalacia.

## Decortication

Decortications have been performed on 43 patients, 24 men and 19 women, who have been followed for between 3–6 years. There were 76% good or very good results and 24% poor results. There was a slight deterioration with time in 8 cases. The majority of these were treated by patellectomy but the reason for the failure remains uncertain in two cases. In the remainder, the main cause seems to have been the poor functional quality of the newly formed tissue. The prognosis is, we think determined largely by the postoperative management. Nevertheless, these figures must be considered encouraging, particularly in view of the severity of the cartilage changes which almost always included ulceration on both sides of the joint. In conclusion, I would remind the reader that the surgery of the chondromalacia is essentially a surgery of the pain and, therefore, always keeps a bit of mystery.

**References**

1. Bandi W: Chondromalacia patellae and femoro-patellare arthrose. *Helvet Chir Acta* (Suppl. II):70, 1972.
2. Ficat P: *Cartilage et Arthrose.* Paris, Masson, 1978, p 120.
3. Ficat P, Ficat C, Gedeon P, et al: Spongialization. *Clin Orthop* 144:74, 1979.
4. Ficat P, Hungerford D: *Disorders of the Patello-Femoral Joint.* Baltimore, Williams & Wilkins, 1978, p 264.
5. Ficat P, Hungerford D, Philippe J: Chondromalacia patellae. A system of classification. *Clin Orthop* 144:52, 1979,
6. Ficat P, Philippe J: Contrast arthrography of the synovial joint. New York, Masson U.S.A., 1981, p 172.
7. Maquet P: Biomechanics and osteoarthrosis of the knee. XIeme SICOT Congress, Mexico, 1969, Bruxelles 1970.
8. Vivalta V, Moya J, Mora Y, et al: Condrografia femoro rotuliana. *Rev Orthop Traum* 211 B, 1978.

CHAPTER NINE

# Proximal Realignment in the Treatment of Patellofemoral Pain

JOHN N. INSALL, F.R.C.S.

The majority of us believe that there are several causes for the syndrome of anterior knee pain. One of the most important subgroups is that associated with malalignment. Other causes of anterior knee pain will not be included in this discussion. Among the criteria used in the diagnosis of this condition are an increase in the quadriceps angle causing the patella to ride against the lateral lip of the patellar groove and patella alta or high-riding patella which may be associated with subluxation. Each variation may result in abnormal patellar tracking due to lateral deviation of the patella when the extensor muscle contracts (5) (Fig. 9.1A and B).

In the diagnosis of patella alta there are a number of methods used, nearly all of them radiographic (7). The one that we use and have found most satisfactory is based on the fact that in a normal knee joint the diagonal length of the patella and the length of the patella tendon are equal (Fig. 9.2). This measurement can be made independent of the position of the knee as long it is in slight flexion to take up any slack in the patellar tendon. The patellar tendon must be measured to the tibial tubercle and if it is 1 cm or longer than the diagonal length of the patella, then there is a high-riding patella (6).

The quadriceps angle is the normal valgus angle between the pull of the quadriceps and the alignment of the patellar ligament (Fig. 9.3). It is a clinical measurement and cannot be determined radiographically. Such a clinical measurement is open to some error but often one can make this observation from across the room. If the patient stands with the feet together, one may see the patellae facing inward, the characteristic "squinting of the" patellae (8) and as Professor Ficat et al. (3) have reported, this is

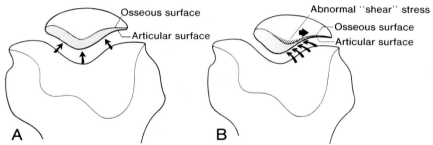

**Figure 9.1.**   A (*left*). A normally situated patella without malalignment. The articular pressure is distributed evenly from the surface. B (*right*). Lateral tracking of the patella creates an uneven distribution of the surface pressure which results in 1) deformation of the cartilage of the vertical crest and 2) abnormal shear stress and intensified loading in the subchondral bone which may exceed the pain threshold. It should be recognized that this can occur even when the articular surface is intact. Reprinted with permission from Insall et al., *Clin Orthop* 144:65, 1979 (5).

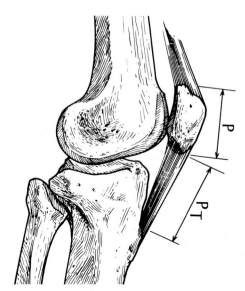

**Figure 9.2.**   Patella alta. Measurements are made on a lateral roentgenogram in the manner shown. Normally the lengths of the patella and patella tendon are equal. When the tendon length exceeds the patellar length by more than 15% (for practical purposes, by more than 1 cm) the patella is high-riding. Reprinted with permission from Insall et al., *J Bone Joint Surg* 58-A:2, 1976.

in fact a combination producing malalignment (Fig. 9.4). It is internal torsion of the femur with compensatory external torsion of the tibia, the result being that the axis of the knee joint is not the same as the hip and ankle.

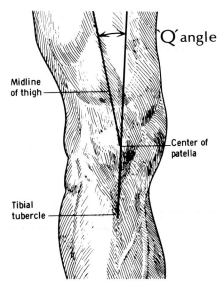

**Figure 9.3.** The Q-angle. See text. Reprinted with permission from Insall et al., *J Bone Joint Surg* 58-A:2, 1976.

Doctor Laurin et al. (9) have described their method for accessing patellar-femoral congruence. We use a similar method, one that was described by Merchant et al. (10). Their technique is to place a patient on a frame with the angle of flexion of the knees at 45°. We use 35°. The x-ray tube is placed proximal to the knee inclined at 30° to the horizontal and the cassette is placed upon the tibia. If correctly carried out, an axial view with the patella in profile is obtained, it must not be blurred nor have any surface superimposed upon another. From this, certain measurements are obtained. First of all is an assessment of the sulcus angle. This is the depth of the trochlea groove. It is obtained by drawing lines from the highest points on the medial and femoral condyles to the lowest point of the intercondylar sulcus (Fig. 9.5). The sulcus angle in the center at point A is then bisected to establish a reference line and a second line is then drawn from the apex of the sulcus angle to the lowest point on the middle articular ridge of the patella. It is then possible to determine the position of the patellar crest in relation to the middle line and the angle between these is a congruence angle. The position of the patellar crest is normally medial and if so, the angle is designated as negative. If the position is lateral, the

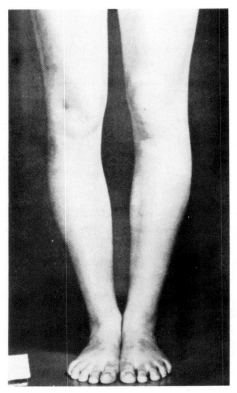

**Figure 9.4.** Squinting knee caps. This type of knee is prone to chondromalacia. The deformities are: 1) increased femoral anteversion, 2) increased Q-angle, and 3) external tibial torsion. As a result, when the patient stands with the feet together, the knee caps face inward. Reprinted with permission from Insall et al., *J Bone Joint Surg* 58-A:7, 1976.

angle is positive and it is abnormal. In order to give you certain parameters of normal measurements, it is necessary to consider some definite numbers. This work was done in Italy by Aglietti and Cerulli (1) and, after measuring 150 volunteers whose knees were asymptomatic, they found the following: the normal Q-angle was 15°. The length of the patella and the patella ligament was equal, being the same. The sulcus angle was 137° and the average congruence angle was −8 with a ±6 tolerance. Aglietti also examined in a similar manner, 90 symptomatic knees, 53 of these are what he called "chondromalacia" where the patient's primary complaint was anterior knee pain. The other

47 were those whose primary complaint was subluxation of the patella and in these he found that the Q-angle was normal but there was a great increase in the length of the patellar tendon. The sulcus was also dysplastic meaning that it was flatter than normal and there was a grossly abnormal congruence angle. Those whose primary complaint was of knee pain, on the other hand, had a statistically significant increase in the quadriceps angle. They had a normal patella and a normal sulcus angle, but there was also an abnormal congruence angle.

In summary, in the patients with subluxation, the patella was high riding, the patella and the sulcus were dysplastic, and the congruence angle was grossly abnormal. In those who complained only of pain, the anatomical abnormality was an increase in the true angle. Thus, in the squinting kneecap, there would also be an abnormal congruence due to imperfect or abnormal patellar tracking and a lateral deviation of the patella contributing to uneven distribution of surface pressure. These findings are, therefore, exactly the same as those found, using a different method, by Carroll Laurin et al. (9).

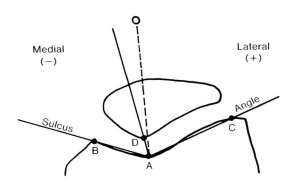

The Congruence Angle

**Figure 9.5.** To measure the congruence angle: Find the highest point of the medial (B) and lateral (C) condyles and the lowest point of the intercondylar sulcus (A). (A clear plastic straight-edge is helpful.) The angle, BAC, is the sulcus angle. Bisect the sulcus angle to establish the zero reference line, AO. Find the lowest point on the articular ridge of the patella (D). (A straight-edge held parallel to the horizontal axis of the patella helps.) Project line AD. The angle DAO is the congruence angle. All values medial to the zero reference line AO are designated as minus and those lateral, as plus. Mean = −6°; standard deviation = 11°. Reprinted with permission from Merchant et al., *J Bone Joint Surg* 56-A:1391, 1974 (9).

This has important implications when one is deciding what to do for the patient. One must demonstrate malalignment by these means before considering an operation for it. The realignment procedure is not appropriate for other causes. Unfortunately, it is impossible to give precise indications for surgery at times, but it should be emphasized that one should not operate on many of these patients. If one is operating on 10% of the patients that are seen with malalignment syndrome, it is probably too many. Most of these patients will have had problems for years before they are considered for surgery. They must have had at least 6 months of continuous symptoms affecting everyday activity, not just when they attempt to play a particular sport and they must have a lengthy period of adequate conservative treatment, exercise, bracing, aspirin, and so forth.

The procedure that is recommended and will be discussed in detail is proximal realignment. Proximal realignment in our experience is indicated when there is patellar malalignment or malposition and it is usually not appropriate when pain is secondary to hyperactivity or direct trauma (5). Distal realignment may produce a short-term result, however, the consequences of transfering the tibia tubercle are all too often productive of late osteoarthritis which is due to a drastic disturbance in the extensor mechanism increasing articular stress (2, 4). Proximal realignment is, therefore, the preferred method for treating these conditions. It consists of a modified quadriceps plasty changing the direction of the quadriceps tendon pull and not changing the tibial tubercle.

The surgical technique is to approach through an adequate straight skin incision (5). The skin flaps are dissected medially and laterally to expose the quadriceps tendon and the borders of the patella. An incision is then made along the border of the vastus medialis crossing the medial quarter of the patella and extending distally to the level of the tibial tubercle (Figs. 9.6–9.8). The second incision is made laterally extending into the vastus lateralis, of the same length as the medial incision. The expansion is dissected from the medial border of the patella and the joint is opened on the medial side. The synovium is removed from the region because this flap is going to be overlapped across the patellar tendon. This results in the vastus medialis together

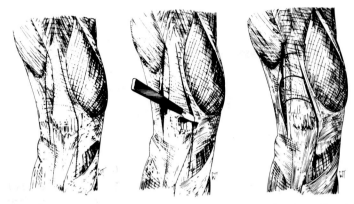

**Figure 9.6.** Line of incisions made in the extensor mechanism. Reprinted with permission from Insall et al., *Clin Orthop* 144:65, 1979 (5).

**Figure 9.7.** The medial third of the quadriceps expansion is separated sharply from the patella to produce a medial "flap." The lateral incision extends into the vastus lateralis muscle and includes the synovial lining. Reprinted with permission from Insall et al., *Clin Orthop* 144:65, 1979 (5).

**Figure 9.8.** The quadriceps "tube" is formed by suturing the free edge of the vastus medialis to the free edge of the vastus lateralis. Reprinted with permission from Insall et al., *Clin Orthop* 144:65, 1979 (5).

with the medial flap separated from the rectus femoris tendon and laterally the insertion of the vastus lateralis into the tendon and adjoining portion of the patella has been divided. It is not, however, a lateral release and medial plication of the capsule. It is a rearrangement of the attachments of the quadriceps tendon. The vastus medialis is brought laterally and distally as far as it will go and the first suture is placed at the upper border of the patella (Fig. 9.9). The second suture at the lower border and then the remaining sutures in the line to form a flattened tube proximal to the patella (Fig. 9.10). The amount of overlap will vary and, in some patients, especially those with marked lateral displacement of the patella, the medial flap may be too large and there is an excessive amount of it. Because this extends completely across the patella, it has been found most satisfactory to roll this flap on itself to remove the slack and suture the edge into a line so that the whole bulk is across the top of the patella. This admittedly produces a rather bizarre appearance and a bulky ridge across the top of the patella. It really looks very much like a breed of dog known as "Rhodesian Ridgeback." The

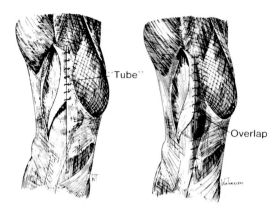

**Figure 9.9.** Approximately at the level of the superior pole of the patella, further suturing causes the patella to rotate medially and the lateral facet begins to lose contact with the femoral condyle. Realignment is sufficient and the tube complete. Reprinted with permission from Insall et al., *Clin Orthop* 144:65, 1979 (5).

**Figure 9.10.** The remaining part of the medial flap is sutured as it lies without further overlap. The suture line is approximately midline and remains stable when the knee is flexed. Reprinted with permission from Insall et al., *Clin Orthop* 144:65, 1979 (5).

excessive tissue, however, disappears very rapidly and it will not be noticed for a very long period of time. It is necessary to do this, however, to restore the balance and this operation has been performed for more than 10 years.

Recently, 75 patients have been examined and one-half of these had a follow-up of more than 4 years. They were all seen at the hospital by one of my colleagues. The anatomical abnormality was the squinting knee, with increased Q-angle in 36, patella alta in 21, and a combination of deformity in 18. In analyzing the results, an excellent knee needs no qualification as it is a relatively normal knee. These patients are able to do anything and have no complaints. A good result had unlimited activity and the patient was able to do anything he desired, but did have some trivial symptoms in the way of pain and some crepitus or loss of flexion. Those with fair results continued to have some pain and symptoms from the knee. Of the 55, 50 were clinically excellent or good and the congruence angle measured postoperatively in this group was −11. The 5 failures, on the other hand, all demonstrated residual incongruence, with an average congruence angle postoperatively of +5. This

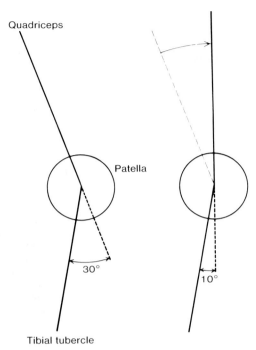

**Figure 9.11.** Diagram showing how proximal realignment influences patellar tracking even though anatomic relationship between patella and femur may actually remain unchanged. Reprinted with permission from Insall et al., *Clin Orthop* 144:65, 1979 (5).

group demonstrated rather nicely that if you leave residual incongruence you have failed the purpose of your operation and the result will be unsatisfactory, either because of persistent pain or persistent instability. If, on the other hand, you restore congruence of the patella and the trochlea, the results are almost uniformly good (5) (Fig. 9.11). Nothing has been said (today) about the articular lesions and the finding in this group were inconstant. About one-half of them had cartilage damage and one-half did not. The treatment over the 10-year period has also varied. Early, the cartilage was shaved or excised but in recent years, this has not been done. The defects have been allowed to remain and it seems to make little difference whether a cartilage lesion when present was shaved or whether it was left alone. We are convinced that in the early lesions of cartilage that they can be allowed to remain without impairing the results of treatment by proximal realignment. In fact, some of the latest results suggest that they may improve. Since our excellent and good results amount to 90.9% of the total number of patients treated, we believe that this is the recommended procedure at the present time.

### References

1. Aglietti P, Cerulli G: Chondromalacia and recurrent subluxation of the patella: A study of malalignment with some indications for radiography. *Ital J Orthop Traumatol* 5:187, 1979.
2. Crosby EB, Insall I: Late results of Hauser procedure. *J Bone Joint Surg* 57-A:1027, 1975.
3. Ficat RP, Hungerford DS: *Disorders of the Patello-Femoral Joint.* Baltimore, Williams & Wilkins Co, 1977.
4. Fielding JW, Liebler WA, Urs D, et al: Tibial tubercle transfer: A long range follow-up study. *J Bone Joint Surg* 56-A:1315, 1974.
5. Insall J, Bullough PG, Burstein AH: Proximal "tube" realignment of the patella for chondromalacia patellae. *Clin Orthop* 144:63, 1979.
6. Insall J, Goldberg V, Salvati E: Recurrent dislocation and the high riding patella. *Clin Orthop* 88:61, 1972.
7. Insall J, Salvati E: Patella position in the normal knee joint. *Radiology* 101:101, 1971.
8. Insall J, Falvo KE, Wise DW: Chondromalacia patellae. *J Bone Joint Surg* 58-A:1–8 1976.
9. Laurin C, Dussault R, Levesque HP: The tangential x-ray investigation of the patello-femoral joint. *Clin Orthop* 114:16, 1979.
10. Merchant AC, Merek RL, Jacobson RH, et al: Roentgenographic analysis of patello-femoral congruence. *J Bone Joint Surg* 56-A:1391, 1974.

# CHAPTER TEN

# Osteoarthritis of the Patellofemoral Joint: Anterior Displacement of the Tibial Tuberosity

**PAUL MAQUET, M.D.**

In describing the patellofemoral joint, we must keep in mind the forces acting on the joint (2) (Fig. 10.1). To flex the knee, the force $F$ acts with a lever arm $e$, the origin of which is the axis of flexion of the femoro-tibial joint. The moment $F.e$ is counterbalanced by the force $P_a$ exerted by the patella tendon acting with the lever arm $c$ which has the same origin as $e$. The two moments $F.e$ and $P_a.c$ are equal. The femoro-tibial joint transmits the force $R$ which is the resultant force of $F$ and $P_a$. This same force $P_a$ acts on the patellofemoral joint with a completely different lever arm $k$, the origin of which is the center of curvature of the weight-bearing surfaces of the patellofemoral joint. The moment $Pa.k$ is equal to the moment $M_v.q$, q being the lever arm of the force $M_v$ developed by the quadriceps tendon. The two lever arms $k$ and $q$ here again have the same origin. The force applying the patella against the femur is the resultant $R_5$ of $M_v$ and $P_a$. This force changes during flexion of the knee. The force $R_5$ becomes greater and greater with flexion. The two forces $P_a$ and $M_v$ cannot be equal since their lever arms $k$ and $q$ are different. When the lever arms change, the forces must change as well in such a way that their moments remain equal. The force $R_5$ is transmitted from the patella to the femur, the weight-bearing surfaces of which have been measured by Townsend et al. (8). These weight-bearing surfaces increase and move upward on the patella from full extension to 90° flexion. Transmitted through these weight-bearing surfaces, the force $R_5$ causes compressive stresses in the joint.

These stresses appear in the x-rays. As Pauwels (7) has shown,

123

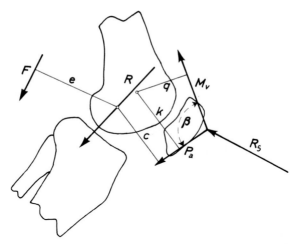

**Figure 10.1.**   Sagittal projection of the forces acting on the knee. $F$ = force tending to flex the knee; $e$ = lever arm of force $F$; $P_a$ = force exerted by the patella tendon; $c$ = lever arm of force $P_a$ acting on the femoro-tibial joint; $k$ = lever arm of force $P_a$ acting on the patellofemoral joint; $M_v$ = force exerted by the quadriceps tendon; $q$ = lever arm of force $M_v$; $R$ resultant of forces $F$ and $P_a$; $R_5$ resultant of forces $M_v$ and $P_a$.

everywhere in the skeleton the quantity of bone depends on the magnitude of the stresses and the subchondral sclerosis presents exactly the same outline as the diagram of the stresses in the joint. In the normal joint, subchondral sclerosis has the same thickness throughout: the stresses are evenly distributed. If the subchondral sclerosis is cup-shaped with a maximum of thickness in the middle, the stresses are unevenly distributed and are increased compared to normal. An increase of the subchondral sclerosis means an increase of the stresses. If we consider the normal joint projected on a coronal plane, the quadriceps pull $M_v$ forms an angle with the pull $P_a$ of the patella (Fig. 10.2). The resultant force $R_5$ of $M_v$ and $P_a$ is directed laterally. The possible causes of an increase of force $R_5$ in this projection are easy to determine. If the leg is in valgus and the other parameters remain normal, the closing of the lateral angle between the femur and the tibia will increase the length of this vector. Force $R_5$, thus, will be increased by the valgus deformity of the leg. An abnormal lateral position of the tibial tuberosity will have the same effect. By closing the lateral angle, formed by the two forces $M_v$ and $P_a$, this lateral position of the tuberosity increases the force $R_5$. If the vastus medialis is weaker than normal, the pull of $M_v$ will be misdirected in such a way that $R_5$ becomes also increased.

Figure 10.1 showed a sagittal projection and Figure 10.2 shows a coronal projection (4). In Figure 10.3, a transverse projection of the patella is represented by the skyline view. In this x-ray, the subchondral sclerosis is practically of even thickness throughout. This means that the stresses are evenly distributed over all articular surfaces and, therefore, each facet must transmit a component of $R_5$ proportional to its area: $R_L$, the lateral component of $R_5$, is greater than $R_M$, the medial component of $F_5$. This may be demonstrated on photoelastic models. Certain materials, when loaded, become birefringent. The model represents a cross-sectional model of the knee. If the load acting on the model is directed as $R_5$ is normally directed, isochromatics of the same order appear behind the two facets. If the patella is subluxated laterally, the medial part of the joint can no longer transmit the load which has to be transmitted solely by the lateral compartment of the joint. This increases and distributes

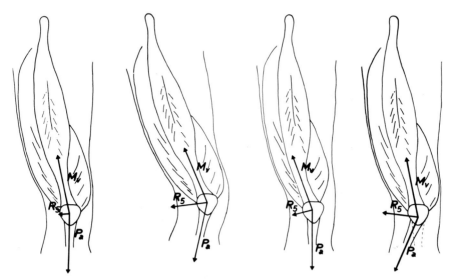

**Figure 10.2.** Coronal projection of the forces acting on the patellofemoral joint. $M_v$ = force exerted by the quadriceps tendon; $P_a$ = force exerted by the patella tendon; $R_5$ = resultant of forces $M_v$ and $P_a$.

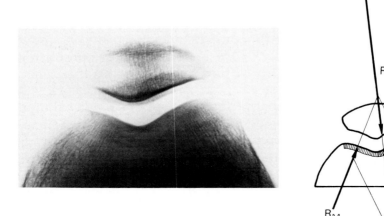

**Figure 10.3.** Horizontal projection of the forces acting on the patellofemoral joint. $R_5$ = patello-femoral compressive force; $R_M$ = medial component of $R_5$; $R_L$ = lateral component of $R_5$.

unevenly the stresses in the joint. When the patella of the model is subluxated, the isochromatics attain a much higher order. This means that the stresses are much greater than they were in the normal model. This change may be read in the x-rays. The subchondral sclerosis becomes cup-shaped and thicker beneath the lateral facet of the patella. This demonstrates that the stresses are concentrated and abnormally increased in the lateral aspect of the joint. The medial facet and the medial aspect of the patella are stressed less than normally. The medial subchondral sclerosis and the underlying cancellous bone fade away.

It is interesting to compare the different stages of osteoarthritis of the patellofemoral joint (Fig. 10.4). The two facets of a normal patella are underlined by a subchondral sclerosis of even thickness throughout (Fig. 10.4A). This means an even distribution of the compressive stresses in the joint. A cup-shaped subchondral sclerosis under the lateral facet demonstrates an increase and an uneven distribution of the compressive stresses (Fig. 10.4B). This may represent the very first sign of patellofemoral osteoarthritis. Subjected to abnormally high stresses, the cartilage disappears while the thickness of the subchondral sclerosis increases and the normal structure of the cancellous bone in the medial aspect of the patella tends to disappear (Fig. 10.4C). Finally, even the bone no longer can withstand the exaggerated stressing and is resorbed (Fig. 10.4D). Osteoarthritis, thus, appears as a breakdown of the equilibrium which normally exists between the resistance and the mechanical stressing of the tissues. A simple and final solution to this problem consists of removing the patella. Considering again a sagittal projection of the knee (Fig. 10.1), the patella provides the force $P_a$ with a lever arm $c$. The compressive force transmitted from the femur to the tibia is the resultant force $R$ of $P_a$ and $F$, $F$ representing the flexing forces. If we remove the patella, the tendon falls into the intercondylar groove, shortening the lever arm of the force $P_a$. To carry out its work, the quadriceps has to develop a much greater force and the resultant force $R$ is considerably increased.

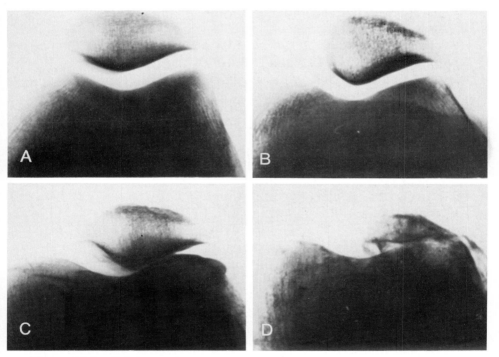

**Figure 10.4.**   Subchondral sclerosis corresponding to the stress diagram. A. Normal knee. B. Cup-shaped sclerosis, first sign of osteoarthritis. C. Cup-shaped sclerosis and narrowing of the joint space. D. Destruction of bone.

Thus, patellectomy has solved the problem of patellofemoral osteoarthritis but has created a problem in the femoro-tibial joint. It seems more sensible to attack the cause of osteoarthritis, the disturbance of equilibrium between resistance and stresses in the tissues of the joint. Since we can hardly change the resistance of the tissues, there remains only one solution. This consists of decreasing the compressive stresses in the joint. These compressive stresses or articular pressure can be reduced either by diminishing the force which is transmitted across the joint or by enlarging the load transmitting surfaces of the latter. The ideal consists of combining both possibilities, decreasing the load and enlarging the load-bearing surfaces. We can decrease the pressure in the joint by recentering the subluxated patella into the intercondylar groove, through a lateral retinacular release. This enlarges the load-bearing surfaces of the joint. However, if there is osteoarthritis or if the osteoarthritic patella is not subluxated, the retinacular release does not seem to be sufficient.

I suggest displacing the tibial tuberosity anteriorly (3, 5). The operation lengthens the lever arm $c$ of the force $P_a$. Thus, the patellar tendon can carry out its work by transmitting a smaller force. But above all, this anterior displacement opens the angle formed by the two forces $M_v$, quadriceps tendon, and $P_a$, patella tendon. Even without changing the magnitude of these forces, just opening the angle as occurs in an anterior displacement by 2 cm will reduce $R_5$ by about 50%. This may be demonstrated in a geometric analysis of all the forces acting on the leg during gait. Anterior displacement of the tibial tuberosity by 2 cm decreases the patellofemoral force $R_5$ by 50% and decreases the femoro-tibial force $R_4$. These forces were also calculated for the first phases of the unilateral support period of gait when the quadriceps is acting. From the calculation it also appears that an anterior displacement of the tibial tuberosity by 2 cm would reduce by about 10% the force $P_a$ exerted by the patella tendon. It would reduce to less than 50% the compressive force $R_5$ transmitted from the patella to the femur.

The operation is very simple. The incision is medial, 12–15 cm long about 1 cm behind the tibial crest and parallel to it. Holes are drilled transversely behind the tibial crest to mark the osteotomy line and then the osteotomy is completed either with a saw or a chisel. The whole crest is raised with the tuberosity and it is maintained in this position by inserting an iliac graft on edge at the upper extremity of the osteotomy. The only problem may be the skin in some cases. I do not hesitate to carry out medial and lateral relieving incisions to avoid tension on the skin. The patient can move immediately. He walks and returns to work after some weeks.

Figure 10.5 shows a 53-year-old lady who complained of a very painful knee with a limitation of the movements. A thick, cup-shaped subchondral sclerosis was present in the patella. A considerable anterior displacement of the tibial tuberosity (2.5–3 cm) was carried out. Immediately the pain disappeared. The knee regained a full range of movement. The structure of the

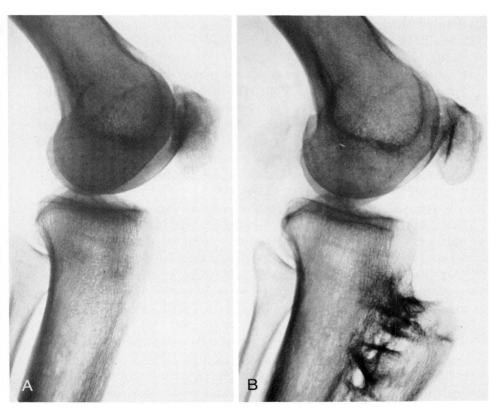

**Figure 10.5.**  A 53-year-old female patient before (A) and 6 years after a sufficient anterior displacement of the tibial tuberosity (B).

cancellous bone and the subchondral sclerosis dramatically changed. These changes demonstrate that the pressure has been reduced in the joint and that the compressive stresses are now evenly distributed. The follow-up period is 6 years.

The cosmetic appearance may be an inconvenience. A photograph showing the anterior bulge is shown to the patients, who have to decide whether the relief of the pain they experience is worth the deformity. Usually they do not hesitate when they are at this stage.

If the patella is subluxated, it is not sufficient to decrease the load transmitted from the patella to the femur, but we must also enlarge the articular weight-bearing surfaces by recentering the patella into the intercondylar groove. This may be achieved by displacing the tibial tuberosity anteriorly and medially. Notches are cut in the graft which will maintain the tibial tuberosity displaced anteriorly and medially.

In the painful knee of a 43-year-old male patient (Fig. 10.6), the patella was subluxated laterally. The cup-shaped subchondral sclerosis again indicates an increase of the joint pressure. After a marked anterior (3 cm) and medial displacement of the tibial tuberosity, the pain disappeared. The range of movement became normal. The patient walked normally. The patella has been recentered and the change in its structure is apparent. The thin ribbon of subchondral sclerosis now shows that the stresses are evenly distributed and considerably decreased in relation to what they were before the operation.

We have just reviewed a series of patients essentially from two orthopaedic centers (6). The ages range from 15 to 88 years with a maximum of cases between 55 and 68 years. The follow-up was between 1 and 10 years. The effect on pain was spectacular. Before surgery, all patients experienced pain. After surgery, most of them reported no pain at all or some slight pain when overusing the knee. The range of movement remained good or was improved. We observed a change for the better in the structure of the cancellous bone and the subchondral sclerosis. We tried to find out how much anterior displacement was necessary to achieve a good result. There were fewer poor results with further advancement of the tuberosity. The maximum of good results was achieved for an anterior displacement of the tuberosity by 26 mm and more (Fig. 10.7).

In order to study postoperative changes, systematic arthros-

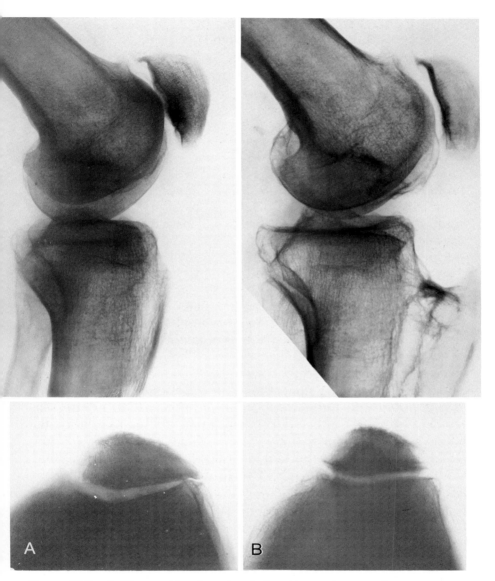

**Figure 10.6.** A 43-year-old male patient before (A) and 5 years after a sufficient anterior and medial displacement of the tibial tuberosity (B).

copy has been carried out in such cases before and after anterior displacement of the tibial tuberosity, by Fujisawa et al. (1).

Before surgery, the load-bearing surfaces are constituted of eburnated bone. This is replaced by a covering of white bright

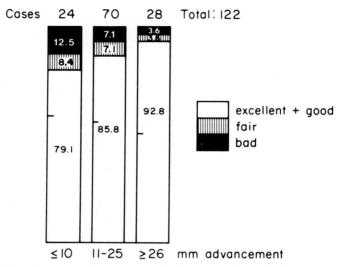

**Figure 10.7.** The percentage of excellent and good results increases with the importance of the anterior displacement of the tibial tuberosity.

tissue after some months. This tissue seems to have improved in quality at later follow-up. Actually, Fujisawa et al. (1) show pictures of fibrocartilage with a tendency of the deep layers to become hyaline. But if the anterior displacement is not sufficient, the patella ends up with a crab meat kind of cartilage.

When we carry out a barrel vault osteotomy of the tibia for medial osteoarthritis of the knee, we used to displace the distal fragment anteriorly, even if there is no patellofemoral osteoarthritis, since the anterior displacement of the tuberosity decreases the load transmitted from the femur to the tibia as well as the force transmitted from the patella to the femur. We have used the same approach to treat painful knees following patellectomy with or without lack of extension.

Thus, it is possible to read the distribution of the articular stresses in the x-rays. It is also possible surgically to improve the distribution of the stresses in the patellofemoral joint in order to achieve a therapeutic effect. This leads usually to a regression of the signs of osteoarthritis.

## References

1. Fujisawa Y, Masuhara K, Matsumoto N, et al: *Arthroscopy* (Japanese) 3:56, 1978.
2. Maquet P: *Biomechanics of the Knee.* Berlin, Heidelberg, New York, Springer Verlag, 1976.
3. Maquet P: Considérations biomécaniques sur l'arthrose du genou. Un traitement biomécanique de l'arthrose fémoro-patellaire. L'avancement du tendon rotulien. *Rev Rhum* 30:779, 1963.
4. Maquet P: Rappel biomécanique. In: Déséquilibre et chondropathies de la rotule. *Rev Chir Orthop* 66:209, 1980.
5. Maquet P: The biomechanics of the knee and surgical possibilities of healing osteoarthritic joints. *Clin Orthop* 146:102, 1980.
6. Maquet P, Watillon M, Burny F, et al: Traitement chirurgical conservateur de l'arthrose du genou. *Acta Orthop Belg* 48:204, 1982.
7. Pauwels F: *Biomechanics of the Locomotor Apparatus.* Berlin, Heidelberg, New York, Springer Verlag, 1976.
8. Townsend PR, Rose RM, Radin EL, et al: The biomechanics of the human patella and its implication for chondromalacia. *J Biomech* 10:403, 1977.

# CHAPTER ELEVEN

# Chondromalacia: Treatment Based on a More Precise Diagnosis*

**ERIC L. RADIN, M.D.**

First, let me put into perspective what others have said. It has been made very clear that there is no direct relationship between the histological state of the cartilage lesion and the patient's symptoms. Since articular cartilage has no nerves, patellofemoral pain comes from either synovial inflammation or increased nervous pressure in the underlying bone (5). It has become apparent that a fibrillated area of articular cartilage on the patella will not necessarily progress into an arthrotic lesion. As was shown initially by Meachim and Emery (9), fibrillated cartilage can survive. With the advent of arthroscopy, many of us have been able to follow cartilage lesions in our patients over time and have observed absolutely no progression of most medial facet lesions. Ward Casscells, among others, has beautifully documented this in a very large and well-studied series of patients (3). However, in contrast to lesions on the medial facet, there is a strong tendency for the cartilage lesions on the lateral facet to progress to bare bone (10). Everyone agrees that as you grow older the cartilage changes tend to spread.

This distinction between lesions which have a tendency to progress or not to progress (to bare bone) is terribly important in treating patients. There is no reason to treat cartilage lesions that are not going to progress.

If one defines chondromalacia as cartilage softening and fibrillation, then the term has pathological significance but not clinical significance. The problem in the patella is that we can have lesions which tend to progress and which do not tend to progress side by side. On the medial side, we generally have an

* This work was supported by NIH grant AM27127.

earlier onset of cartilage lesions which tend not to progress; on the lateral side, cartilage lesions tend to occur at a later age and frequently spread to eventually involve the entire patella (Fig. 11.1). Contact studies have shown that both facets bear load so that nonprogression on the medial area is not the result of nonweight-bearing (16). Rather, it probably has something to do with the nature of the bone. The bone under the medial facet is

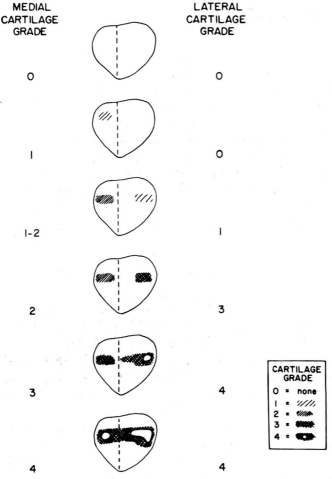

**Figure 11.1.** Lesions which originate in the medial side usually do not progress to Grade IV (bare bone) Collins lesions. Cartilage damage which initiates on the lateral side will progress and can spread to cover the medial side. Reprinted with permission from Abernethy et al., *J Bone Joint Surg* 60-B:205, 1978 (1).

less dense and less well ordered than under the lateral facet, most apparent in a frontal view (Fig. 11.2) (1). The trabecular pattern of bone in the medial central area is disordered in all patellae, whereas there was a very pronounced reproducible trabecular pattern in the normal patella over the rest of the patellae (4). If one looks at the bone and its relative stiffness area by area, a stiffness map can be generated (Fig. 11.3). This shows that the bone in the medial central facet is relatively osteopenic and there is more normal, denser, stiffer bone on the lateral side and under the crest (15). Because of this, there is a sharp stiffness gradient or change in stiffness on the medial side of the crest. This is the region where the initial cartilage changes occur. One of the initiators of cartilage fibrillation can be a steep stiffness gradient in the underlying bony bed (13). The explanation for that is that cartilage will fibrillate if you subject it to a tensile stress (Fig. 11.4). If you want to rip something apart, pull on it. If there is a relative difference in bony compression, there will be a concentration of tensile strain in the cartilage overlying that area of steep gradient in the underlying bony stiffness.

"Chondromalacia" should be thought of as a nonprogressive, limited, age-related cartilage deterioration or degeneration not

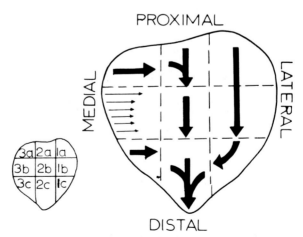

**Figure 11.2.**   Frontal view of the patella showing the prominent orientation of the trabecular bone. Note that the medial central facet has no prominent orientation. Reprinted with permission from Townsend et al., *J Biomed Mater Res Symp* 7:608, 1976.

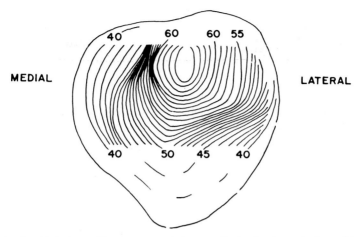

MEDIAL                                                                    LATERAL

**Figure 11.3.**   Relative stiffness map of the patella in the frontal plane. Note that the bone in the medial facet is less dense than that on the lateral side. Reprinted with permission from Abernethy et al., *J Bone Joint Surg* 60-B:205, 1978 (1).

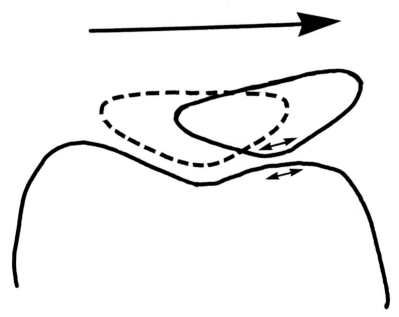

**Figure 11.4.**   In order to fibrillate, cartilage must be subjected to a tensile stress so that it is "torn." An example of how such stress is applied to cartilage is by subluxation of the patella.

associated with symptoms and occurring in the central medial facet area (12). Its presence at arthrotomy should be treated as an incidental finding. This lesion does not cause pain. It is universal and certainly everyone does not have patellofemoral or anterior knee pain.

The initiation and progression of cartilage lesions must be two distinct phenomena (11). Fibrillation does not necessarily progress. All of us, at the time of total knee replacement, have seen patellae which are absolutely devoid of articular cartilage. When one looks at the progressive patellar lesions as they spread, they do indeed move from lateral to medial. Bone tends to get stiffer as the cartilage lesions progress (1, 11). This tends to suggest that the state of the underlying bone and the pressure distribution on the lateral side are playing some role in this.

Chondromalacia, then, is a pathological term but not a meaningful clinical term. If chondromalacia, clinically, is defined as anterior knee pain, then it is a generic term like internal derangement of the knee. In my view, much of the confusion and controversy surrounding chondromalacia of the patella is that many orthopedic surgeons try to treat clinical chondromalacia (anterior knee pain) as a disease without appreciating that anterior knee pain is the result of a variety of conditions. We should either stop using the term clinically or realize that clinical chondromalacia has subsets, such as patellofemoral osteoarthrosis, osteochondral lesions, subluxation of the patella, etc. There has been some confusion about the definition of malalignment. Maldague (8), an orthopaedic radiologist, has shown that in taking patellar skyline x-rays it makes a difference whether the quadriceps is contracted or not. He showed that if the quadriceps is contracted, what looks like a subluxed patella will be moved back into the patellar groove (8). A question logically can be raised as to how significant "patellar malalignment" measurements are when they are based on x-rays taken when the quadriceps is not contracted (Fig. 11.5).

Who should be considered a surgical candidate? Realignment procedures should never be done prophylactically. Pain is the only indication for such surgery. Drs. Ficat (Chapter 8) and Maquet (Chapter 10) have both shown, in their presentations, that hypertrophy and sclerosis occurs on the lateral side and over the central crest in patients with pain. Something is going

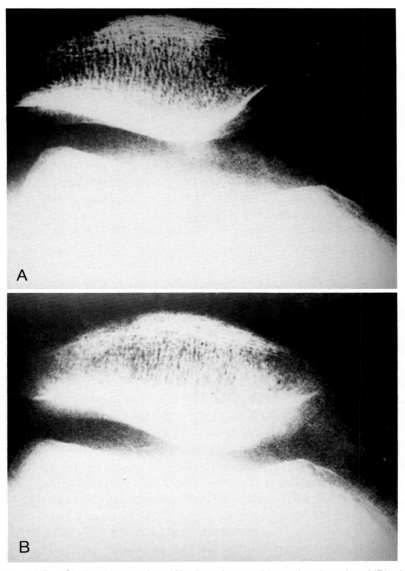

**Figure 11.5.**   Skyline views taken (A) when the quadriceps is relaxed and (B) when the quadriceps is tightened. Note that the patella tends to migrate laterally when the quadriceps is relaxed and springs back into the groove when the quadriceps is contracted. Reprinted with permission from Maldague and Malghem, *Acta Rheum Belg* 1:109, 1977 (8).

on in the bone. The bone is related to the cartilage change and the bone is clearly related to the pain. Maquet (Chapter 10) has shown in his work that when the bone changes go away, the pain goes away.

Now, I would like to say something about the cartilage healing. You have heard many of the panel say that they pay absolutely no attention to the state of the cartilage lesions. Dr. Maquet (Chapter 10), for example, says he does not even look in the knee joint. He bases his surgery on whether he thinks there is hyperpressure or not. Professor Ficat (5) does look at knee joints arthrographically, but also primarily bases his surgery on localization of tenderness and not on the nature of the lesion. I would like, for just a few moments, to review an experiment we did several years ago (14). We did not do it on patellae, we did it on the hips. However, it proves the point that cartilage can heal functionally and stay healed if the pressure on it is reduced. What we did was to remove the articular cartilage of the hip joint and the acetabulum of a group of cats, and then sacrifice them at various times after that. One-half of the cats underwent a hanging hip procedure. A hanging hip procedure is multiple tenotomies about the hip (14). Described by Voss, it unloads the hip about 25%. Two and one-half years after removal of all the articular cartilage in an animal who had its muscles reattached, the hip articulates an eburnated bone and there are osteophytes (Fig. 11.6). The acetabulum is cobblestone in appearance. This is similar to the sort of hips that we do total hip procedures on. The hanging hip cats healed their joints with fibrocartilage and without evidence of osteoarthrosis. As Professor Lemperg pointed out (Chapter 5), reconstitution of hyaline cartilage, a very sophisticated and specialized structure, should not be expected. One hopes to achieve functional healing in the patients.

Metaplasia to cartilage from cells other than condrocytes can occur in fracture callus or pseudoarthrosis, for example. Hyaline cartilage can develop. There is good clinical evidence that cartilage metaplasias occur after osteotomy, and Mr. Goodfellow (6) and others have published photographs of fibrocartilage and, indeed, hyaline-looking cartilage forming after osteotomy, as has the Mayo Clinic Group (Personal Communication). After hanging hip procedures done on patients with congruent hip joints and joint space narrowing, the joint space came back (14). Now

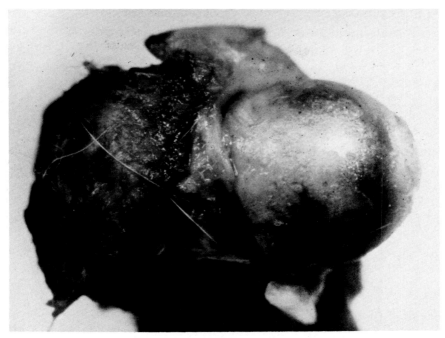

**Figure 11.6.**  Appearance of the femoral head of a cat 2½ years after total removal of the articular cartilage and a hanging hip procedure. Note the reformation of a chondroid surface. The control hip, which had all of its cartilage removed but no muscle releases was severely osteoarthrotic at the end of the same time period. Reprinted with permission from Radin et al., *Clin Orthop* 112:221, 1975 (14).

the Japanese are looking arthroscopically after osteotomy and finding lesions actually healing (7), not healing with normal hyaline cartilage but healing with fibrocartilage.

For healing, one must follow three rules (2): 1) there must be motion; 2) a source of cells must exist to provide the healing; 3) a situation of diminished pressure must be created. Synovium is an excellent source of cells for metaplasia to cartilage. Fortunately, the patella is totally surrounded by synovium. If you have no synovium overgrowing and the bone is dense and eburnated, the argument for multiple drillings or whatever you want to call it, spongialization, can be made and one can obtain cartilage forming from these drill holes or curettage holes. Professor Ficat's lateral release (Chapter 8) and Professor Maquet's anterior tibial tubercle advancement (Chapter 10), both reduce the pressure across the patellofemoral joint and allow such healing tissue to last.

Probably the worst thing that can be done in the immediate postoperative period is to increase the pressure by demanding repeated straight leg raising. That is highly stressful to the knee joint, and is something that should not be allowed in the immediate postoperative period. Of course, control of the leg is desired, but passive motion rather than active motion might be the goal in the immediate several weeks at least.

The experience with just drilling cartilage lesions on the patella has been dismal in most hands. It is not necessary, as has been discussed by several of our faculty. They have had excellent results totally ignoring the cartilage surface. If one is dealing with a fairly large laterally or centrally placed lesion and feels obligated to drill, go ahead, as long as the pressure is also reduced. On the medial side of the patella, it is not necessary.

I might conclude with a word about cartilage shaving. The argument is that one must go in there and shave off fibrillations because they will contribute to a synovitis. This has not been borne out clinically. Fibrillation on the medial side does not usually tend to progress. Effusion in patients with anterior knee pain is not common. This means that there is usually not much synovial inflammation. The articular shaver is probably one of the most misused instruments that we have available today.

I would like to make two further comments. One is just to re-emphasize that the pain cannot be related directly to the cartilage lesion and the second is, as Dr. Casscells has pointed out (Chapter 7), we are excessively arthroscoping our patients with patellofemoral discomfort. As you heard from Professor Ficat earlier (Chapter 8) and from Carroll Laurin during the earlier discussion (Chapter 6), one cannot really tell which patients are going to do well with conservative management. It has been our experience that most of them do well. There is no reason to perform a big battery of diagnostic procedures or a relatively expensive arthroscopy unless the patient is refractory to conservative management. Therefore, the pressure to make a specific diagnosis is not really necessary unless the patients do not get better by themselves. I generally allow my patients 3 months, and I cannot tell you whether the progressive resistance exercises I order strengthen the quadriceps or realign the patella. I believe that both probably do occur in some percentage of cases. I concur with what Dr. Hungerford (Chapter 6) stressed, that using Sybex and Nautilus machines is not reasonable physical therapy. On reasonable physical therapy, most of these patients will get better by themselves. If they do not, then the search for diagnosis is essential.

### References

1. Abernethy PJ, Townsend P, Rose RM, et al: Is chondromalacia patella a separate entity? *J Bone Joint Surg* 60-B:205, 1978.
2. Akeson W, Miyashita C, Taylor TKF, et al.: Experimental arthroplasty of the canine hip. *J Bone Joint Surg* 51-A:149, 1969.
3. Casscells W: Gross pathological changes in the knee joint of the aged individual. *Clin Orthop* 132:225, 1978.
4. Darracott J, Vernon-Roberts B: The bony changes in "chondromalacia patella." *Rheumatol Phys Med* 11:175, 1971.
5. Ficat P, Hungerford DS: *Disorders of the Patello-Femoral Joint.* Baltimore, Williams & Wilkins, 1977.
6. Macys JR, Bullough P, Goodfellow J: Resurfacing of femoral head after osteotomy: A report of three cases. *Clin Orthop* 123:143, 1977.
7. Koshino T: The treatment of spontaneous osteonecrosis of the knee by high tibial osteotomy with and without bone-grafting or drilling of the lesion. *J Bone Joint Surg* 64-A:47, 1982.
8. Maldague B, Malghem J: Chondromalacia patellae: A radiological approach. *Acta Rheum Belg* 1:109, 1977.
9. Meachim G, Emery IH: Cartilage fibrillation in shoulder and hip joints of Liverpool necropsies. *J Anat* 116:161, 1973.
10. Meachim G, Emery IH: Surface morphology and topography of patello-femoral cartilage fibrillation in Liverpool necropsies. *J Anat* 116:103, 1973.
11. Pedely RB, Meachim G: Topographical variation in patellar subarticular calcified tissue density. *J Anat* 128:737, 1979.
12. Radin EL: A rational approach to the treatment of patello-femoral pain. *Clin Orthop* 144:107, 1979.
13. Radin EL, Abernethy PJ, Townsend P, et al: The role of bone changes in the degeneration of articular cartilage in osteoarthrosis. *Acta Orthop Belg* 44:55, 1978.
14. Radin EL, Maquet P, Parker H: Rationale and indications for the "hanging hip" procedure: a clinical and experimental study. *Clin Orthop* 112:221, 1975.
15. Raux P, Townsend PR, Miegel R, et al: Trabecular architecture of the human patella. *J Biomech* 8:1, 1975.
16. Townsend PR, Rose RM, Radin EL, et al: The biomechanics of the human patella and its implications for chondromalacia. *J Biomech* 10:403, 1977.

# CHAPTER TWELVE

# Panel Discussion: Can We Successfully Treat Chondromalacia of the Patella?

**MODERATOR, JOHN GOODFELLOW, M.S., F.R.C.S.**

**Moderator:** "Dr. Casscells, do you allow your patients who have had adolescent anterior knee pain to play sports after their symptoms have disappeared?"

**Dr. Casscells:** "I'm not against it if they are young. I feel more secure if it is a female rather than a male in returning to full athletics, perhaps because males tend to engage in more competitive athletics and in contact sports."

**Moderator:** "Carroll Laurin?"

**Dr. Laurin:** "Sports never destroy a knee. However, patients should respect their pain which is a signal. I'm against it if there is malalignment. If there is muscle imbalance, I think it is necessary to work on the vastus medialis to build it up."

**Moderator:** "Eric Radin?"

**Dr. Radin:** "I think one has to adjust one's activity levels to avoid pain. I allow activity as long as it remains asymptomatic."

**Moderator:** "John Insall?"

**Dr. Insall:** "I make a decision as to the cause of the pain. If I believe it is from overuse, such as jogging, I recommend giving that activity up."

**Moderator:** "David Hungerford?"

**Dr. Hungerford:** "I'm against returning to activities. Quadriceps exercise increases resistance and if you have changes in the patellar cartilage, it is not a good idea."

**Moderator:** "I wouldn't think myself that this would become indicated if the pain is not too severe after athletics. Let me ask the panel what they would do for anterior knee pain in patients who have normal x-rays."

**Dr. Laurin:** "I would do a parapatellar block with xylocaine. Pain relief lasts longer than the physiological duration of the anesthetic agent."

**Dr. Hungerford:** "The question of symptoms from the patello-femoral joint is completely unresolved. I think that recurrent malalignment may give only symptoms at the time of the transient malalignment as a sense of knee instability. This may take decades to produce symptomatic cartilage degeneration. From the work of Ficat and Philippie, we know that there is radiological evidence of malalignment fairly frequently in the opposite asymptomatic knee of patients presenting with a symptomatic knee, that is, the x-ray of both knees are abnormal but only one knee is symptomatic. We are all well versed in the quotation, "we don't treat x-rays", but I think we also have to be aware of the fact that normal x-rays can be seen in the presence of some pretty significant degenerative changes, and that these normal x-rays may not be representative of the situation that the patellofemoral joint may be occupying in heavy use, particularly running, twisting, and turning. TNS is sometimes helpful. I would not inject the knee."

**Dr. Radin:** "I would try to find the cause of the symptoms although I must admit that initially I will treat the younger patients with quadriceps strengthening exercises for 6 weeks and in 90% of the patients, that usually works. It is not until I have had a failure of conservative treatment that I even consider arthroscoping the patient."

**Dr. Casscells:** "I surprisingly find myself in total agreement with Dr. Radin. I think too many arthroscopic examinations are carried out for weak indications."

**Dr. Insall:** "It is necessary to check around the tendon particularly below the patella and see if one can find a trigger point. It is surprising how many of the patients in this category have patellar pain without patellar cartilage lesions and really have patellar ligament difficulty."

**Moderator:** "Dr. Lemperg?"

**Dr. Lemperg:** "Since anterior knee pain is a symptom and not a definite pathophysiological entity, it appears that attempts to clarify the source of pain is an important step. Among other causes that should be considered is the syndrome associated with interosseous hypertension. In the presence of normal x-rays, the diagnosis can be made in a patient with a history of pain at rest—aggravated by activity, by determining the interosseous pressure—note prolonged drainage there and by increased activity in a Technetium bone scan. Intra-articular changes including synovitis may be excluded by arthroscopy. If no specific findings can be reached, a repeat examination after appropriate time should be made in order not to overlook a bone tumor."

**Moderator:** "Professor Ficat?"

**Dr. Ficat:** "Axial views and arthrography as well as analysis of synovial fluid can be very helpful. We prefer the single contrast dye technique for arthrography in those. Though we have difficulty distinguishing these initially 50% of the patients will be better without surgery. If there is a cartilage lesion we try lateral retinacular release. There is no way to decide about those who will get better conservatively. Our indications for lateral release is increased pressure on the lateral side. This is manifested by tenderness with patella pressure over the lateral side of the patella, narrowing of the joint space laterally on properly taken axial view and increase in subchondral sclerosis on the lateral side."

**Dr. Laurin:** "I find myself in agreement with Professor Ficat, that I am unable to predict who is going to do well with conservative treatment ahead of time. More extensive investigation is done including new x-rays and repeat examinations are continued until we have a more exact diagnosis. The term chondromalacia of the patella is not a diagnosis any more than osteoarthrosis is a diagnosis. We must know the exact type of difficulty in order to obtain a more satisfactory result."

**Dr. Insall:** "I agree as well. With malalignment, patients probably do better with proximal realignment than with any other form of treatment."

**Moderator:** "What about distal realignment?"

**Dr. Insall:** "The Hauser procedure produces other incongruent changes, for example, the relationship of the tibia in rotation. Many patients develop patellofemoral osteoarthrosis after 5 or 10 years. One can relieve lateral pressure but it may increase the overall patellar pressure."

**Dr. Hungerford:** "The important thing in doing a tibial tubercle-plasty is not to move the tibial tubercle too far in any direction. This is accomplished best by a coronal osteotomy similar to that proposed by Bandi for tibial tubercle elevation. This gives you a flat surface in which to rotate the tibial tubercle medially and also very slightly distally. In so doing, the tibial tubercle is not depressed posteriorly which is biomechanically bad. I think that the tendency to lift off a block of the tibial tubercle and move it a long way distally and medially, but also a long way posteriorly because it was implanted into the metaphysis was a biomechanically unsound procedure. If the coronal osteotomy is carried out then the tubercle can be fixed with K wires and it is not necessary to immobilize the knee. Also the tubercle can be moved 5 or 6 mm, fixed temporarily, the knee put through a range of motion to check on patella tracking, and then move it another few millimeters if it is thought to be necessary. I have used this type of tibial tubercle-plasty since 1974 and I have never needed to immobilize the knee or had one pull off."

**Moderator:** "What are your indications, Dr. Maquet, for tibial tubercle advancement?"

**Dr. Maquet:** "Painful osteoarthrosis of the patello-femoral joint of patients who complain of painful patellofemoral joints and their double contrast arthrograms demonstrate fissures or other significant cartilage lesions."

**Moderator:** "Have you ever arthroscoped your patients pre-operatively?"

**Dr.Maquet:** "Yes, that can replace the double contrast arthrogram as a valuable diagnostic tool."

**Moderator:** "How do you treat your patients postoperatively?"

**Dr. Maquet:** "I ask them to move immediately. They are allowed full weight-bearing on the leg and walk."

**Moderator:** "How quickly do they walk?"

**Dr. Maquet:** "From the 2nd day."

**Moderator:** "Dr. Maquet, what are the complications of anterior tubercle advancement?"

**Dr. Maquet:** "Skin necrosis and difficulty in kneeling. The skin necrosis can either come from too tight a dressing or too much pressure under the skin. We have seen both. I show patients who are candidates for anterior tibial tubercle advancement a photograph of what it looks like ahead of time and discuss with them that they may have difficulty kneeling postoperatively."

**Dr. Hungerford:** "We have some experiments to show that the Maquet procedure of the anterior tibial tubercle advancement actually increases the contact area of the patellofemoral joint. Thus, the result may not be due purely to dimunition in overall force but the two factors."

**Moderator:** "Dr. Maquet, do you wish to comment?"

**Dr. Maquet:** "That is very interesting and I would very much like to see the data."

**Moderator:** "Dr. Insall, do you have other comments about distal realignment?"

**Dr. Insall:** "I believe that the degree of correction of the incongruence would be directly related to the relief of pain postoperatively. Also, cartilage improved or became asymptomatic after realignment. If osteoarthrosis occurs with bare bone, realignment cannot be successful, then something else must be done."

**Dr. Hungerford:** "If distal realignment is associated with increased pain, it is very often because the distal realignment has been overdone or the tibial tubercle has been implanted deep into the medial metaphysis so that the patellar tendon is coming into conflict with the anterior margin of the tibia as the knee flexes and the patella sinks into the intercondylar notch. This can be corrected by anterior displacement of the tubercle with a bone block as described by Maquet and Bandi. In fact, this is very similar to the problem that arises from the patient with patellectomy and the treatment is the same."

**Dr. Laurin:** "One should also consider incongruity iatrogenically, such as postmeniscectomy."

**Moderator:** "Is there any advantage to patellar splints?"

**Dr. Hungerford:** "I have personally tried several patellar braces and have not found any of them to be very effective. I think that the superficial braces such as an ace wrap and some of the other soft braces simply provide a cutaneous stimulus which gives the patient a much greater cerebral awareness of his knee and can, therefore, protect it better with voluntary restriction of the movement that causes symptoms."

**Moderator:** "Is surgery indicated in young persons whose growth plates are not closed?"

**Dr. Insall:** "Yes, if they are habitual patella dislocators and, in that case, surgery certainly should be of the soft tissue itself."

**Moderator:** "Dr. Laurin, do patients with complete loss of articular cartilage (bare bone) have knee pain and what percentage of individuals?"

**Dr. Laurin:** "Occasionally, particularly if there is also malalignment."

**Moderator:** "Have you ever advocated or tried osteotomy of the patella as a method to relieve pain?"

**Dr. Laurin:** "Yes, for patellofemoral osteoarthritis but not for chondromalacia patella."

**Moderator:** "Dr. Lemperg, do individuals with patellofemoral osteoarthritis have pain more frequently than those with rheumatoid arthritis?"

**Dr. Lemperg:** "Pain at rest is rather uncommon in rheumatoid arthritis but most patients have discomfort with motion."

**Moderator:** "Do you have any preconceived numbers as to what percentage of patients with anterior knee pain do not have either malalignment or patella alta?"

**Dr. Laurin:** "About 20%. Malalignment occasionally can produce these symptoms but must be demonstrated before doing anything corrective."

**Dr. Hungerford:** "We have just completed some biomechanical studies on patella alta and have found that moving the tibial tubercle distally is, in fact, biomechanically a sound procedure. The contact area is actually increased by distal tibial tubercle transplantation given the degree of knee flexion and although such distal movement results in a slightly increased quadriceps force needed to extend the knee, this is offset by the increased contact surface and the unit load for articular cartilage is reduced. Patella alta is often associated with patellofemoral instability and so, therefore, if distal realignment is necessary, it can be coupled by medial and distal realignment."

**Moderator:** "Does anyone believe that patellectomy produces an increase in the possibility of tibiofemoral osteoarthritis?"

**Dr. Laurin:** "Not tibiofemoral osteoarthritis, but it does not solve the problem and probably should never be done for chondromalacia patella."

**Moderator:** "Dr. Laurin, do you recommend the Maquet procedure and if so, will you give us your indication?"

**Dr. Laurin:** "Yes, in combination with realignment if there is also malalignment. The chief indication is when other procedures have failed."

**Moderator:** "Dr. Maquet, have you used anterior tibial tubercle advancement for patients with patellectomy?"

**Dr. Maquet:** "Yes, in these cases I insist that the advancement be at least 2 cm and preferentially more, as much as possible as indicated."

**Moderator:** "Why?"

**Dr. Maquet:** "It is a matter of lever arms. You have to compensate for the absence of the patella which requires more than just improving the leverage of an existing patella."

**Moderator:** "Have you ever had any skin complication?"

**Dr. Maquet:** "Yes."

**Moderator:** "How do you treat it?"

**Dr. Maquet:** "Dakins solution and waiting, they take a long time to heal."

**Moderator:** "Have you ever had osteomyelitis secondary to the skin complications?"

**Dr. Maquet:** "Yes, I removed the graft once. The advancement fortunately persisted and the patient had relief of the anterior knee pain."

**Moderator:** "Some have suggested that the tibial tubercle only needs to be advanced 1½ cm and that that can be done through a transverse incision. What is your comment?"

**Dr. Maquet:** "Burke and Ahmad (*Proc ORS*, 1980) show that the more you do, the better it is. They were up to 3 cm of anterior displacement. None of the authros that claimed 1–1½ cm is enough have ever published the postoperative patient's changes and the structure of the subchondral bone. I published postoperative x-rays showing the changes in the bone are evident only after significant advancement. On the other hand, I have seen such patients who have had limited displacement and they keep complaining. I have carried out an additional anterior displacement and the complaints have stopped. The pain disappeared."

**Moderator:** "Some claim that the success of the Maquet procedure depends on what lateral retinacular release is done. What is your thought?"

**Dr. Maquet:** "I have performed lateral retinacular release in a few patients without success. The percentage of lasting good results after lateral retinacular release also is disappointingly low. We have reviewed the results of anterior tibial tubercle advancement from several centers with follow-up at 5 years and more and the majority of these patients remain as good results. Furthermore, I do not believe I have performed a complete retinacular release when I do an anterior tubercle advancement through a medial incision."

**Moderator:** "How many of the patients with anterior displacement do not complain?"

**Dr. Maquet:** "It depends upon how sure you want to be about your results. But I would not bet on the future of patients who keep subchondral alterations in their patella postoperatively. If you are doing anterior tubercle advancement in patients who have no subchondral bony changes then you are operating on patients who, in my opinion, have no indications for such surgery."

**Moderator:** "Dr. Radin, you do not seem to like exercise programs for the patellofemoral joint in young persons."

**Dr. Radin:** "Yes, since straight leg raising is stressful to the patellofemoral joint, it would seem that anterior knee pain in adolescent females has nothing to do with the patellofemoral joint but must be some problem with soft tissue. The problem is that they may be better by building the strength of the quadriceps which one assumes must be preferential to the vastus medius. Thus, those patients may well be suffering a subclinical form of malalignment which could be corrected by quadriceps strengthening. I have no other explanation but, certainly, if it was a cartilaginous or a subchondral lesion, straight leg raising would make it more uncomfortable. We do see that straight leg raising is very painful in patients who have cartilage lesions such as following a osteochondral fracture or osteoarthritis."

**Dr. Hungerford:** "In straight leg raising, the articular cartilage usually involved is not in contact so I tend to use isometric exercises and do not have as much difficulty as Dr. Radin says he is having."

**Dr. Radin:** "Refractory joints require diagnostic efforts and treatment if indicated. If you have done something to a knee cap and it does not get better, you must continue with your diagnostic procedures whether you are more comfortable with arthroscopy or arthrography until you really know what is going on."

**Dr. Hungerford:** "It is also pretty difficult to tell what the role of minor subluxations may be in producing articular cartilage lesions. However, if at arthroscopy one sees articular cartilage damage located to that area of the patella which comes into high pressure contact with subluxation, then I think we are only justified in doing either a lateral release or, if there was also an increased Q-angle, perhaps a tibial tubercle-plasty as well. If the area was circumscribed in full thickness, it might also be worthwhile to do a chondrectomy by which I mean a vertical excision of the involved area with drilling of the base."

**Moderator:** "Increased stress on the cruciates may well increase tibial-femoral compression."

**Dr. Hungerford:** "Dysplasias of the trochlea and dysplasias of the patella are major problems that I do not believe can be solved by surgery. If you have lateral subluxation with erosion of the trochlear articular cartilage, I think that this can be treated by a Pridie procedure of simply drilling the sclerotic bone. This is a similar procedure as that which is done for the patella and it seems to be effective. It also has been mentioned that extreme rotation malalignments, that occur only rarely, may require correction."

**Moderator:** "To summarize briefly the thoughts presented today, we may state:

Anterior knee pain presents because of a variety of entities.

Chondromalacia patella is a waste basket term as used clinically. Strickly speaking chondromalacia patella is a pathological diagnosis of an asymptomatic cartilage change.

Careful history and physical examination aided by x-rays and arthroscopic examination should disclose a reasonable basis for the diagnosis and treatment of anterior knee pain.

# Index